Stem Cell and Platelet Therapy

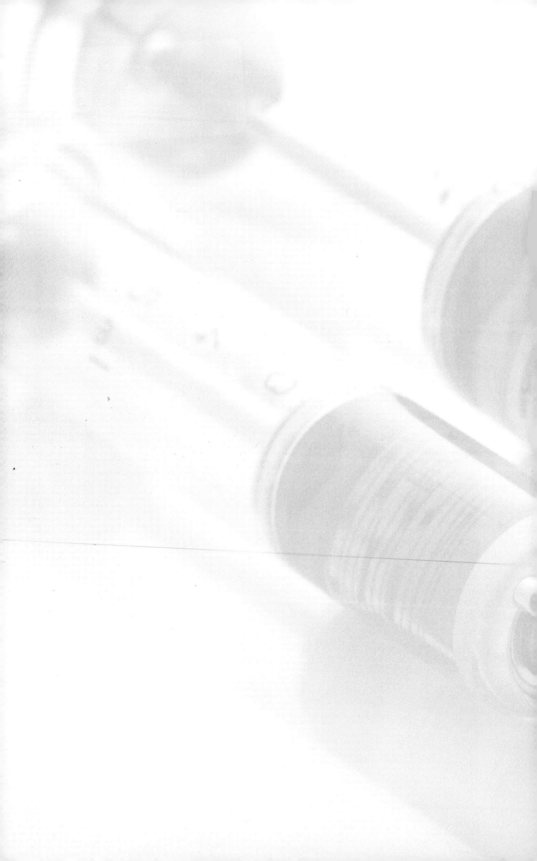

Stem Cell and Platelet Therapy

Regenerate, Don't Operate

MARC DARROW, MD, JD

PROTEX PRESS

PUBLISHED BY PROTEX PRESS

IMPORTANT NOTE: This book is not a substitute for medical advice from your doctor. The general principles presented here may not apply to your medical condition, and they may even be harmful to you. Before embarking on an exercise program or changing your diet substantially, please consult a medical doctor.

DISCLAIMER: Neither Dr. Darrow, nor any associate, is engaged in rendering professional medical advice or services to the individual reader. This information is offered for educational purposes only. Do not act or rely upon this information without seeking independent professional medical advice. This information does not create a physician-patient relationship nor guarantees the accuracy, completeness, usefulness or adequacy of any resource, information, apparatus, product, or process available from this book.

First edition

ISBN: 978-0-9714503-5-6

Book design by Tanya Maiboroda

Acknowledgments

Thanks to Barry Weiner for working with me on this book and many other projects for so many years. You have never failed me, nor let me down.

ALTHOUGH I WANTED to be a doctor since I can remember, I didn't study enough in college, and let medical school pass me by. Instead I went to law school without any specific goal, and wasn't planning on practicing law. Then I met John-Roger (J-R), who told me I was going to be his lawyer, live with him, and be on his staff. The temptation fueled my discipline to study, and I passed the bar exam on the first try using an organizational method that he taught me. During the long weeks of the Bar review course, I was awakened at 5 am to his screaming at me in my head, "Get the hell out of bed and study." (He was in Los Angeles, and I was in Berkeley). At the age of 40, after practicing law for 15 years for J-R and my own practice, J-R told me it was now time to go to medical school. I had a successful practice, and good life as a lawyer. I had built a large house with a gym and 70-foot lap pool down the center in Mandeville Canyon near J-R's house, but was ready to leave for my dream. He yelled at me in front of a retreat gathering of 100 or so of his students, and told me that I was going to go to medical school, and he didn't care if it was in Mexico, Hawaii, or anywhere else, but I would go. The dean of admissions in Hawaii, James Linman, MD, told me he was going to "save my soul, Son." I hadn't even done Pre-Med. During my med-school interview, Gary

Watabayashi told me that I was admitted, and that my teacher (J-R) had sent me to him. After my second year of medical school, at J-R's Santa Barbara ranch, he told me that my wife was having an affair. He said not to worry because he had another woman waiting for me when I returned. As usual I resisted him, and told him I was too busy in medical school to be with this new woman. I think my words were, "Please don't do that to me." His response was, "It's too late, I can't undo this one."

That was 1992, and the new woman, Michelle, and I have been together since then, with 3 beautiful daughters.

And then there's my mom, who continued to press me to stay in medical school every time I was ready to drop out. "You don't have to be a doctor, but you will finish, and it will build your character." She was pure love.

And Dad, you were always amazing in your support for me every time I screwed up. You never once judged me, but only loved me.

As I look back, there are so many people that I am indebted to. So many who have loved and supported me. You know who you are, and there are too many to list. So let me say thanks to you all, and know that I love you and thank you for being there when I needed you most.

And last, but certainly not least, are my amazing staff. Each of you are special to me, and provide the structure of the healing environment that our patients experience. Your hard work and dedication make my life a breeze, and give me the energy to do this heavenly work. I am so grateful to you. *Aloha nui loa.*

—Marc Darrow, MD, JD

Contents

Why I Love Regenerative Medicine

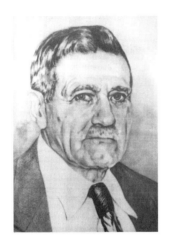

Some of my early memories were being with Edda, my grandfather. Selma, my mother, made sure that I wrote frequent letters to Edda, asking philosophical questions.

Edda always answered these. I have a few that I just pulled out from my desk drawer. The phone on his letterhead is Lafayette 3-6212, and the address is 1811 west 47th Street, Chicago 9.

He wrote to me as if I were an adult, although the dates on these particular letters from him range from when I was 12–14 years old. He used examples of nature to exemplify human character and concepts of life.

He made it clear that he did not follow the crowd, and that a man of wisdom listened to his own heart. One of his mentors said, "If a man does not keep pace with his companions, perhaps it is because he hears a different drummer. Let him step to the music which he hears, however measured or far away" (Henry David Thoreau). And this was always his message to me. I was pounded with opening my mind and seeing things as they are, not as I was told they are. One of his letters states, "Sin is a breach or violation of any rule or statement made by so-called religious authority. So you see there are many sins for there are many holy authorities."

My parents, sibs, and I had lunch at his house frequently. My mom brought the food. As a child and young teenager, I never wanted to go, because I just wanted to play baseball with my friends. Nevertheless, I did respect him, as we all did. To me he was an old wise man, occasionally pounding his fist on the kitchen table when making a point. I remember someone talking about going to Europe, and his fists came alive, and he said, "God Damn It, get your own house in order."

Although he looked and seemed gruff, it never bothered me since he always had a loving smile for me. I will never forget that smile. I was "forced" by my mother, against my will to spend my precious Sundays with him. My mom and I knew I was going to be a doctor, so this was my youthful internship with Eli (Edda) Stenn, MD. He had gallon bottles of cherry syrup, and my job was to pour it into small bottles that he would give to his patients as placebo medicine (As a doctor now, I would always rather use placebo than pharmaceutical medication since placebo has been shown to heal in 30-40% of cases, and pharmaceuticals have been shown to injure and kill in many cases.) Researchers found that America's leading cause of death isn't heart disease or cancer: it's conventional medicine. They found that the iatrogenic death rate in the US (death caused by doctors and/ or medical treatments) is 783,936 a year. To wit, my sister Leila died quickly from a dose of chemotherapy, and not from the cancer that had been surgically excised.

On several Sundays, he would take me to the train station in Chicago, and we would make the trip to Tremont in the Indiana Sand Dunes. Mr. Morgan, his friend, would sometimes come for the trip, and they would discourse on all facets of life. While on our hike one day, they were talking about how powerful man was in relationship to nature, and how man conquered nature. In my boyish manner, I peeped out, "Then why is man afraid to die if he is so powerful. Isn't nature more powerful than man?" Well that really got them going, and then their discussion was about how amazing it is that knowledge is contained in youth, although not normally recognized by adults.

During the same period when I was 12, I was a member of the Great Books Club with my parents at the University of Chicago, and I had plenty to feed Edda and his disciples about Socrates, Plato, Aristotle, ad infinitum. I wasn't really into it, but it was fun to watch their delighted excitement when their new disciple spouted "wisdom." The best part about Tremont was the little store where Edda bought us both a bottle of cream soda, my favorite drink to this day.

I met my Guru (John-Roger) in 1972 and have studied with him to this day. Sometime after I met him, I dreamt that I entered Edda's medical office in his house. The plaque on his desk said, "I complained because I had no shoes, until I met a man who had no feet."

I immediately knew that Edda was in the same line of teachers as John-Roger.

Although John-Roger asked me to become a lawyer, and live with him as one of his staff, I always wanted to be a doctor. After finishing law school, and doing his law work for 15 years, he said that now was the time for me to go to medical school and be his doctor. I had spent years with John-Roger discussing and experimenting with natural medicine, and I knew that would be part of my medical path. He told me I would be doing sports medicine, and I quickly fell in love with that field.

The most important bombshell occurred after injuring my wrist when I was playing golf with John-Roger. It just wouldn't heal. At a medical convention out of desperation I had it injected with Prolotherapy (concentrated sugar water), and it was 50% better the next day. I then injected it myself a few times and have had a pain free wrist for many years. Soon thereafter, I had a failed shoulder surgery, and again self-injected it, and it healed the next day. At this point, I started asking my patients to let me inject their injuries. Soon my practice was mostly Prolotherapy. Years later, the technology advanced to PRP and then Stem Cell injections which you will read about in this book. Of course I have injected myself with PRP for subsequent injuries since dextrose Prolotherapy didn't quite do the job. I do believe PRP and Stem Cells will become the central focus of musculoskeletal medicine with surgery falling by the wayside. And I think Stem Cells will eventually be used to heal most degenerative disease as the research evolves. There are already anecdotal instances reported.

So go forth, and multiply your Stem Cells. Heal now!! I wish you health, wealth, and happiness.

—Marc Darrow, MD, JD

Introduction

"To date, no fully successful treatment for osteoarthritis has been reported. Thus, the development of innovative therapeutic approaches is desperately needed." [1]

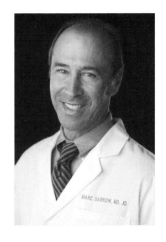

IF YOU ARE reading this, you have most likely come to me, or need to be seen as a patient after suffering from painful and debilitating osteoarthritis or other conditions/injuries involving joints, bones, ligaments, or tendons. You may have been told you have bone-on-bone osteoarthritis and that your only two options are either to have surgery to replace the joint or to just "live with it." It is possible that you have actually had surgery already but have still not experienced relief from your pain.

Based on exciting new research and clinical practice, there is another way. Stem Cell Therapy, Platelet-Rich Plasma (PRP) Therapy, and Prolotherapy injection treatments offer a third, very promising option called regenerative biological medicine. In my office, these treatments are often used in combination. These rapidly evolving technologies mean hope for long-suffering patients and can eliminate the need for surgery, which often does more harm than good. I personally have experienced that.

Medicine is an evolving practice, and the technology of medicine is ever advancing. Tomorrow, Stem Cell Therapy may have evolved into something altogether different as research helps us develop more and better ways to achieve the results we are looking for. In the meantime, continuing research and clinical practice in the areas of Stem Cell Therapy and PRP mean that countless patients can experience relief from pain without the need for surgical intervention. On my weekly radio shows, I use the byline, "Take the Surgery out of Pain."

AT THE DARROW Stem Cell Institute, my goal is to offer an alternative to the "operate or live with it" medical advice most of my patients have received before finding me. It is my hope that this book will give you a greater understanding of these exciting new therapies and arm you with the information you need to make an informed decision about your own treatment. I invite you to contact the Darrow Stem Cell Institute with any questions you may have.

Marc Darrow, MD, JD
Darrow Stem Cell Institute
Los Angeles, CA
800-300-9300
http://www.LAStemCells.com

Foreword

I have known Dr. Marc Darrow of the Darrow Stem Cell Institute for many years. Initially I interviewed him for my book, *Ageless* to find out about his work with regenerative medicine, a natural injection series.

Prolotherapy is an early form of regenerative medicine that has progressed throughout the years to include PRP and Stem Cells.

Regenerative medicine involves injecting a dextrose solution, platelets from the blood, or stem cells and platelets from bone marrow, or just stem cells from fat, into the place where soft tissue is injured, such as the joints, muscles, tendons or ligaments.

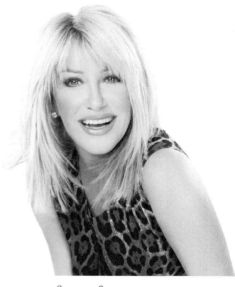

After the interview I was intrigued. I had torn the Meniscus in my right knee while doing my nightly one-woman Broadway show. I went to a surgeon and he recommended surgery. Instead I decided to try working with Dr. Darrow. I was looking for a non-surgical, non-drug way to eliminate the throbbing pain in my knee and I felt we could be a good 'fit'.

Everybody experiences pain at some point in their lifetimes. Our

Suzanne Somers

first pain in life usually happens as kids: we fell off our bikes or other recreational modes and broke our legs and arms. So often later in life these childhood injuries become inflamed 'weak spots' often resulting in dull or whopping, throbbing chronic pain.

Most people with pain pop pain meds and carry on until the meds no longer work. I didn't want to be on drugs so instead I had Dr. Darrow inject his Prolotherapy sugar solution and in time the problem went away, never requiring surgery or pain medications.

Prolotherapy injection is usually paired with a local anesthetic, such as Procaine or Lidocaine. The solution can be sodium morrhuate, sugar or a mixture of sugar and phenol. For my injury, Dr. Darrow gave me a series of injections over a period of about three weeks. I am very happy I chose to be Dr. Darrow's patient. My series of injections worked and surgery was avoided.

Dr. Darrow also treats my son Bruce, an avid cyclist, who has had more 'incidents' than he probably wishes to share with me. But I know each time he has a cycling 'episode' he runs to Dr. Darrow and I feel confident he is with a doctor who is not a pill pusher but rather, solution oriented.

Pain is an overwhelming condition; sometimes so debilitating it destroys happiness and quality of life. Chronic debilitating pain is its own animal . . . and as human beings we will do most anything to eliminate it, thus the rise of prescription pain medications . . . drugs that so often lead to addiction. There is no free lunch with pharmaceuticals and it doesn't take a rocket scientist to know that continued use of heavy duty pain medications is a road to 'no good'.

Dr. Darrow's work has now moved to the new and exciting cutting edge science and breakthrough of stem cell transplants as a therapy. Stem cells are clearly the future and are the better choice instead of surgery which so often brings disappointing results. How many people do you know who had surgery to fix the problem only to have it return, only worse?

Labral tears, bone on bone conditions, degenerative hips, shoulder pain, lower back, disc problems, the list goes on and on.

Pain is ageless. Young people have pain, old people have pain. Athletes have pain so often with injuries that reduce their quality of life. A ballerina friend of mine, once in peak form is now at mid-life, wheel-chair bound. You never know what's going to happen; a serious motorcycle accident or car crash can change your life, a returning veteran with multiple injuries often suffers with life-long debilitating pain. Older people have bones that fracture most often from hormone loss. Testosterone is an anabolic steroid meaning it builds bone and muscle; when testosterone declines the bones decline with it. Estrogen and progesterone also build bone; one burrows, one builds, called osteoclasts and osteoblasts and without hormones you lose this bone building mechanism. This is what you see when an elderly person is crossing the street slowly shuffling. They have no mechanism in place to rebuild lost bones.

But what if you could re-build bone? What if you could eliminate pain permanently? Dr. Darrow understands the effects of bone loss not only related to hormone deficiency but with stem cells rebuilding joint cartilage.

It has long been thought that once bone is gone, it's gone; there's not been much you could do about it, until now. Dr. Darrow asks the question: why not try to first regrow the bone and repair the tissue with the goal of avoiding surgery and eliminating pain?

Isn't this the kind of doctor you are looking for? This book is your opportunity to educate yourself so you can intelligently ask the proper questions and best of all make the right decision for yourself. Surgeons perform surgery. If you go to a surgeon that is what will most-likely be recommended. Most people are not educated about other options. This book offers another option.

Dr. Darrow has been one of the first doctors to use stem cells and Platelet Rich Plasma therapy (PRP). From what I understand he does as much or more of these procedures than any doctor in the world. These treatments come under the term "Regenerative Medicine." Regenerative medicine is the science that studies the regeneration of biological tissues obtained through the use of cells. PRP is obtained from the withdrawal of the patients' blood, concentrating the platelets in a safe, economical way to promote growth factors that stimulate new tissue growth. PRP is able to significantly reduce or eliminate pain and improve joint, tendon, and ligament function.

Science is accelerating at breakneck speed. Both doctors and researchers hope they have found the answer to pain in the promise of bone marrow stem cells. The medical community is excited that stem cells work by rebuilding from within the diseased joint into a healing joint environment. Bone marrow stem cells increase tissue proliferation. Stem cell injections regrow cartilage and stop chronic inflammation. When you have pain, this is what you are looking for.

Before you find yourself addicted to powerful opiates or lying on an operating table with your fingers crossed hoping that this surgery will be the answer to your pain, you now have an exciting new first option; PRP and stem cell therapy might be just what you are looking for. This book could change your life for the better.

—Suzanne Somers

PART ONE

An Introduction to Stem Cell and PRP Therapies

1

The Promise of Stem Cells and Platelet-Rich Plasma Therapies

In my practice, I use stem cells daily to reduce or eliminate patients' pain involving the musculoskeletal system, including but not limited to joints, tendons, ligaments, and muscles from head to toe. The great news is that about 80–90% of patients see improvement with this treatment protocol.

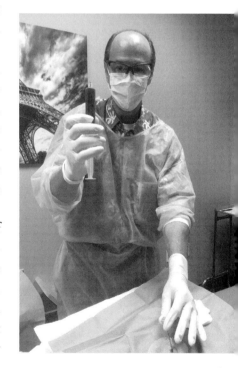

Stem Cell Therapy and Platelet-Rich Plasma (PRP) Therapy are part of a group of treatments that fall under the term "regenerative medicine," which uses the patient's own (autologous) cells to rejuvenate damaged tissues in the body. They are also termed "biomedicine," since they are based on natural biology and chemistry. These therapies do exactly the opposite of surgery: instead of removing damaged tissue, *they rebuild and strengthen it.* They are designed to stimulate the immune system to heal and rebuild damaged joints and tissue without the significant risks that accompany surgery, joint replacement, or

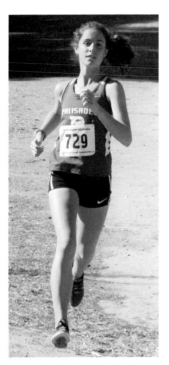

Brittany Darrow

other invasive procedures. I have seen too many infections, instant iatrogenic (doctor caused) arthritis and other injuries, and even deaths as a result of a "simple" surgery.

Patients of all ages and from all walks of life, many sedentary, and many elite athletes, have come to my clinic seeking the pain relief from disability that has eluded them with other treatments. In many cases, these patients have come to me because they are hoping to avoid surgery. I laughingly tell patients that when they go to a barber, they get a haircut; when they go to a surgeon, they get surgery; and when they come to me, they get stem cells and PRP. In my office, we also offer Prolotherapy with dextrose injections for those who request it, but in fact it does not have the healing ability or success of Stem Cell Therapy and Platelet-Rich Plasma (PRP) Therapy. Prolotherapy will be explained briefly below, as will Stem Cell Therapy and PRP Therapy. The latter two, since they are more advanced in their ability to heal, will be discussed in depth in chapters 2 and 3, respectively.

A firm believer in regenerative medicine, I have been using these therapies since 1997, when I was doing my physical medicine residency at UCLA. My Los Angeles clinic, the Darrow Stem Cell Institute, has long been recognized for utilizing advanced, nonsurgical options for musculoskeletal pain, and degenerative joint disease, with Stem Cell Therapy and PRP having become a very exciting option in the past several years. In fact, I have been told by others in my field that no one does anywhere near as much regenerative medicine with Stem Cell Therapy and PRP as I do.

A question I am asked by most patients is why these treatments have never been offered to them by other doctors. Part of the answer to this question is supplied in the research shown below. Despite the availability of evidence-based guidelines for conservative treatment of osteoarthritis, management is often confined to the use of painkillers, physical therapy, surgery, and the wait for eventual total joint replacement. This suggests that many people with osteoarthritis are not made aware of the many different treatments available to them.

I, personally, along with the many thousands of patients I have treated with these techniques since my residency at UCLA, have found regenerative medicine successful in the healing of many parts of the body. In this book, I will share with you the latest medical information on the use of Stem Cell Therapy and PRP for osteoarthritis and soft tissue damage, and I will also present the research supporting their use in the clinical setting for pain in most areas of the musculoskeletal system of the body.

Why Not Surgery?

Many patients have had an arthroscopic surgery, or even multiple surgeries, with less-than-hoped-for results. They are told it is only arthroscopic, and uses small incisions. The truth is that the potential damage is the same. A frequent scenario is something like this: "I had surgery on my left knee, and it made it much worse. I do not want

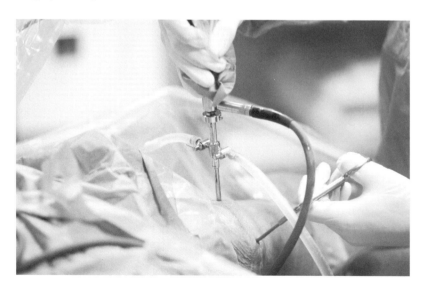

surgery on the right knee!" I hear similar words from patients who come to see me for hip pain or for a variety of other joint, ligament, neck, back, or tendon problems.

A recent article in the *British Medical Journal* addresses the issue of surgery with respect to patients in middle age and above, who represent the largest proportion of those who suffer from osteoarthritis:

> "The benefit of surgery for middle-aged or older patients with persistent knee pain is inconsequential, and such surgery is potentially harmful. Our findings do not support arthroscopic surgery as a treatment for the middle-aged or older person with a painful arthritic knee or torn meniscus."

The article is part of the *British Journal of Medicine's* "Too Much Medicine" campaign that highlights the threat to health and the waste of resources caused by unnecessary care.

Arthroscopic surgery, specifically, is considered to be a waste of resources caused by superfluous care.[2]

When it comes to surgery for treatment of osteoarthritis and other musculoskeletal conditions for patients of ANY age, I am very skeptical, both as a doctor and as a patient. *Surgery should always be the very last option.* The first law of medicine is "Do No Harm". That means when possible, use conservative means, not invasive. In a recent study from Brazil, doctors looked at 510 patients, average age 71 years, who had had either a knee replacement or a hip replacement. One of the findings was a nearly 15% rate of complications.[3]

I see numerous patients of all ages who have had failed surgeries. I myself am an example of such a patient. When I was in medical school, I developed chronic right shoulder pain from a weightlifting injury. After suffering for a year, and having two cortisone injections (I didn't know how destructive they were at the time), my orthopedic surgery professor operated on me. To my great dismay, my shoulder was much worse after the surgery than it had been before. It was swollen, and full of fluid, and I had a fever with blisters near the arthroscopic sites. When I learned about regenerative medicine four years later during my Physical Medicine residency at UCLA, I first had my wrist injected with Prolotherapy, and had a fifty per cent decrease

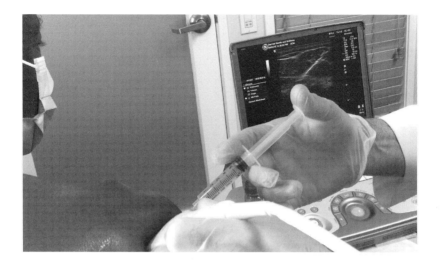

in pain in twenty four hours. After a few more self-injections the pain was gone. I then injected my own shoulder with Prolotherapy, and I experienced complete pain relief just 12 hours later. These self-healings were my wake-up calls. I stopped prescribing pain medications, physical therapy, and surgery, and began to use regenerative medicine to help my patients achieve relief from their pain.

What Is Prolotherapy?

Prolotherapy is the injection of a mild irritant, often dextrose (a simple sugar), into a specific area of the body that is arthritic, worn down, or injured. The newer, far more effective techniques of Stem Cell Therapy and Platelet-Rich Plasma (PRP) Therapy are actually more advanced versions of Prolotherapy, which is short for "proliferation therapy" (the proliferation of new cells following the injection of a substance that will stimulate new tissue growth).

When the irritant is injected into the knee or other area, it causes the body's immune system to stimulate the inflammatory process. While it may seem counterintuitive to create more inflammation, it is in fact inflammation that is part of the body's natural healing response.

This burst of increased inflammation attracts fibroblasts (immature cells present in connective tissue) and chondrocytes (cells that produce cartilage) and brings them to the area of degeneration or injury.

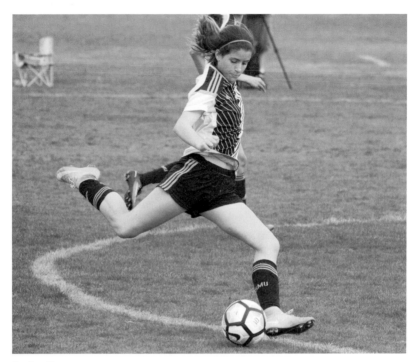

Jordan Darrow

These cells rebuild the collagen (more specifically, what is called the "collagen matrix" of the tissue) and enable it to strengthen and restore the body part in many cases to pre-injury status.

There is a long history of medical studies on the effectiveness of Prolotherapy for knee pain. Recent research done at the University of Wisconsin School of Medicine and Public Health concluded that Prolotherapy resulted in safe, significant, progressive improvement of knee pain, function, and stiffness scores among most participants through a mean follow-up of 2.5 years. The researchers reported that Prolotherapy may be an appropriate therapy for patients with knee osteoarthritis that did not respond to other conservative treatments.

I used Prolotherapy for patients in the past, and at a patient's request rarely employ this technique. The fact is that traditional Prolotherapy has been overtaken by newer, far more effective forms of regenerative medicine, Stem Cell Therapy and Platelet-Rich Plasma (PRP) Therapy. It is these techniques that are shifting the paradigm in the treatment of osteoarthritis and other orthopedics-related conditions. The sections that follow will explain what these therapies are and how they can work for you.

What Is Stem Cell Therapy?

Stem Cell Therapy is the injection of a damaged area of the body with stem cells that have been drawn from the patient's own bone marrow or fat. Stem cells are "de-differentiated pluripotent" cells, which means that they continue to divide to create more stem cells; these eventually "morph" into the tissue needing repair—for our purposes, collagen, bone, and cartilage.

The excitement in the medical community is focused on how stem cells work, rebuilding the damaged part of the body from within by turning a *diseased* joint environment into a *healing* joint environment. Doctors and researchers are hopeful that they have finally found an answer for osteoarthritis in the promise of Stem Cell Therapy.

Numerous studies support the healing effects of stem cells. In one study, doctors tracked patients for five years after they had received stem cell injections for knee osteo-arthritis. At the end of the five-year follow-up period, the knees of patients who had been treated with stem cells were still better than they had been before treatment.[4] At five years, we would have to call that a "curative effect."

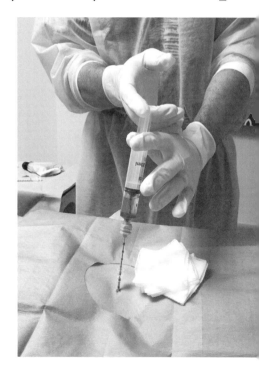

Research has shown that bone marrow stem cells increase the cell proliferation of chondrocytes and inhibit inflammatory activity in osteoarthritis—in other words, according to the researchers, stem cell injections cause the regrowth of cartilage and halt damaging chronic inflammation.[5]

Stem Cell Therapy can be useful not only for the regrowth and repair of cartilage damage, but also for the repair of bone damaged by osteoarthritis. In animal studies conducted in China, doctors found that stem cells injected into the site of a bone fracture promoted rapid and accelerated bone healing.[6]

The research into Stem Cell Therapy has helped revolutionize the way standardized medicine addresses problems of bone degeneration and necrosis (bone death). Cartilage can be regrown, bone can be regrown, and chronic inflammation (swelling) can be shut off.

What Is Platelet-Rich Plasma (PRP) Therapy?

Platelet-Rich Plasma Therapy, or PRP, involves the injection of the damaged area with the patient's own platelet-rich plasma, derived from a blood draw. In 2012, researchers wrote the following regarding the adjuvant use (i.e., assistance in healing after surgery) of PRP:

"Chronic complex musculoskeletal injuries that are slow to heal pose challenges to physicians and researchers alike. Orthobiologics is a relatively new science that involves application of naturally found materials from biological sources (blood platelets and stem cells among them), and offers exciting new possibilities to promote and accelerate bone and soft tissue healing.

Platelet-rich plasma (PRP) is an orthobiologic that has recently gained popularity as an adjuvant treatment for musculoskeletal injuries. It is a volume of fractionated plasma from the patient's own blood that contains platelet concentrate. The

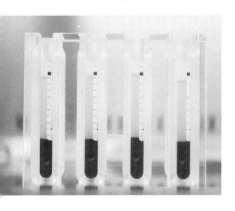

platelets contain alpha granules that are rich in several growth factors that play key roles in tissue repair mechanisms. PRP has found application in diverse surgical fields to enhance bone and soft tissue healing by placing supra-physiological concentrations of autologous [*that is, taken from the patient—author*] platelets at the site of tissue damage. The relative ease of preparation, applicability in the clinical setting, favorable safety profile and possible beneficial outcome make PRP a promising therapeutic approach for future regenerative treatments."[7]

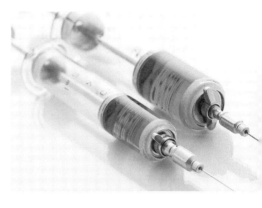

Since that research, numerous studies have noted that PRP has found favor with surgeons in efforts to heal patients' post-surgical damage. Other researchers have demonstrated the benefits of the simpler injection treatment of PRP as a means of avoiding surgery altogether.

Stem Cell and PRP Research at the Darrow Stem Cell Institute

At my clinic, we are currently performing several studies on Stem Cell Therapy and Platelet-Rich Plasma (PRP) therapy.

The Director of Research at my clinic, Brent Shaw, and I, conducted the following research project comparing Stem Cell and PRP therapies in patients suffering from osteoarthritis of the knee, hip and shoulder:

Stem Cell Therapy

Number of Treatments	0	1	2	3
Number of Patients per Treatment	101	101	50	33
Resting Pain (Scale from 0–10)	2.32	1.55	1.20	0.94
Active Pain (Scale from 0–10)	5.91	4.21	3.96	2.82
Total Improvement (Scale from 0–100%)	—	35.48%	43.10%	60.45%
Functionality Score (Scale from 0–40)	20.81	23.92	24.16	27.24

PRP Therapy

Number of Treatments	0	1	2	3
Number of Patients per Treatment	40	40	20	15
Resting Pain (Scale from 0–10)	2.20	1.53	1.45	1.20
Active Pain (Scale from 0–10)	6.30	5.08	4.45	4.02
Total Improvement (Scale from 0–100%)	—	29.28%	32.75%	38.33%
Functionality Score (Scale from 0–40)	22.18	22.65	23.15	24.60

- As seen in the tables above, both treatments have been shown to decrease patient pain as well as show an increase in patient overall improvement and functionality of the joint.
- Consistent with prior research, the Stem Cell Therapy compared to PRP shows a more impactful patient improvement in pain and functionality of the treated osteoarthritic joint.

2

Stem Cell Therapy

In my practice, I use stem cells daily to reduce or eliminate patients' pain involving the musculoskeletal system, including but not limited to joints, tendons, ligaments, and muscles from head to toe. The great news is that most patients see improvement with this treatment protocol.

How Stem Cell Therapy Works

The use of bone marrow-derived stem cells was first tested in the 1960s. Even then, doctors knew that stem cells had unique regenerative powers due to their ability to morph into bone and cartilage and migrate to the site of damage once introduced into the body. Using stem cells from a patient's own bone marrow or adipose (fat) tissue was particularly interesting, because these types of autologous stem cells are readily available without ethical (embryonic) problems in their use. In musculoskeletal

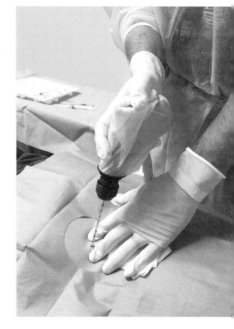

medicine, stem cells provide an answer to the conundrum of cartilage and other soft tissue rejuvenation.

Some research suggests that the introduction of stem cells into the joint also reawakens and revitalizes the stem cells already present in the synovial fluid of the knee, as well as in the cartilage and bone. This "supercharges" the healing process of all structures in and around the joint (cartilage, menisci, ligaments, and tendons).

Stem Cell Therapy is considered a solution with limited side effects.

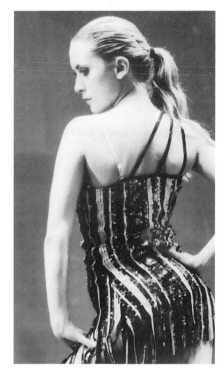

Jensen Darrow

Where Do We Get the Stem Cells for Therapy?

For each treatment, stem cells are taken from the patient's iliac crest at the back of the pelvis. These cells are valuable because they are undifferentiated cells, meaning that they do not have a tissue type but can grow to become other, more specialized types of cells. If a joint, cartilage, tendon, ligament, or muscle needs regeneration, stem cells can supply the building material.

How Is the Procedure Done?

The Stem Cell Therapy injection procedure is a very simple, in-office procedure with no general anesthesia, as it involves almost no pain. Moreover, it takes only about 30 minutes from start to finish. During bone marrow Stem Cell Therapy, a practitioner will inject lidocaine at the top of the buttocks, at or near the posterior superior iliac spine, to numb the area. A tiny incision (which heals quickly after the procedure) is made to allow insertion of a needle to aspirate bone marrow. No stitches are necessary. The solution obtained is spun in a centrifuge. The stem cells are then harvested and injected into the target area or joint under ultrasound guidance when required. Although bone marrow aspiration is typically painful during other procedures such as bone marrow transplantation, it is nearly pain free in this case. A relatively small amount is collected.

Joints: Repairing, Not Replacing

Joint osteoarthritis can involve a myriad of pathologies, among them loss of cartilage, trauma, overuse, postsurgical trauma and tissue removal, bone hypertrophy, metabolic diseases such as gout or pseudogout, and autoimmune diseases such as rheumatoid arthritis, psoriatic arthritis, and infectious destruction. When I see a patient with a previous recommendation for joint replacement surgery, it is usually because traditional medicine considers that the joint is damaged enough that repairing or providing treatment options other than replacement surgery are not practical or warranted.

However, research has clearly shown that Stem Cell Therapy can repair and rebuild bones and the cartilage that covers them. This was documented in a study on diabetic patients in which doctors reported

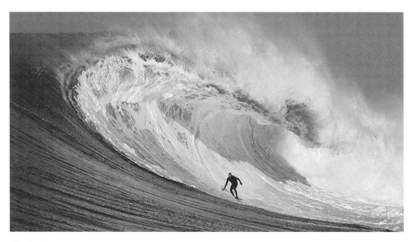

Benjy Darrow

that adding stem cells from human bone marrow to a fractured diabetic bone augmented the repair process and increased the strength of the newly formed bone.

Bones of diabetics are known to be more fragile than those of non-diabetic people and can take longer to heal after a fracture. Diabetics are more likely than non-diabetics to sustain fractures as a result of falling, as they often suffer from impaired vision and reduced sensitivity in their feet.

Bones healed with the addition of Stem Cell Therapy were significantly stronger and able to withstand more stress than the bones of patients in a control group.[8]

Stem Cells Change the Healing Environment

In new research, doctors have found that stem cells work by changing the environment of the joint they are working on—basically, they "turn on the lights" and call in construction crews of helper cells.

Researchers looked at the remodeling and healing done by osteoblasts—specialized mesenchyme-derived (stem) cells accountable for bone synthesis. They found that these cells rebuild bones through various mechanisms, including "cell homing" or "cell signaling."[9] What this means is that the stem cells "communicate" with the surrounding tissue to help them navigate to the site of the wound, then differentiate themselves into bone-building material. Other research suggests positive results even in cases of avascular necrosis (death of bone tissue due to a lack of blood supply), where stem cells were able to sequester blood cells to the site.[10]

This research confirms other studies[11] which speculate that not only could Stem Cell Therapy repair bone damage in cases of hip osteonecrosis (bone death), but it could also halt the disease acceleration by correcting the decrease in the local mesenchymal stem cell populations, reinforcing the natural healing environment.

In preclinical studies, the use of stem cells uniformly demonstrates improvements in osteogenesis (bone formation) and angiogenesis (blood vessel formation).[12] The stem cells modulate the healing environment in a positive manner.

THIS MANIPULATION OF the healing environment extends beyond the bone itself to include the regeneration of cartilage. *Rebuilding cartilage in severe osteoarthritis is considered one of the great challenges in orthopedic medicine.* Stem cells provide a solution to this challenge because they are plentiful, can direct themselves to morph into collagen fibers (cartilage), and are able to modulate the immune response of the microenvironment of the stem cells already present in the diseased tissue.[13]

In other words, the new stem cells *have the ability to change the environment and revitalize the stem cells already present in the diseased joint.*

Which Work Better: Stem Cells from Fat or from Bone Marrow?

The two types of stem cells that have been used in Stem Cell Therapy are adipose (fat) cells and bone-marrow stem cells. At the time

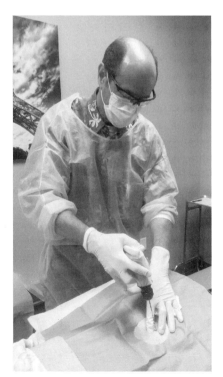

of writing this book, I use bone marrow-derived stem cells because I can better achieve the patient's treatment goals using this approach.

In the past, I have used adipose (fat) stem cells, but I found the use of these cells more traumatic for the patient: in addition to the need to break up fat tissue with a long trocar (an instrument with a sharp point) to obtain the cells, it's necessary to use a thick needle for the injections.

In my experience, not one patient has liked this.

In contrast, bone marrow aspiration (harvesting stem cells

from bone marrow) is nearly painless for most patients after a lidocaine injection and takes only about a minute once I've located the specific area to aspirate. The bone marrow cells can be injected with a very small needle, instead of the larger needle to accommodate the denser fat. In addition, when we use bone marrow, we are injecting both platelet-rich plasma (PRP) from the bone marrow *and* stem cells from the bone marrow—in essence, two treatments instead of one.

Researchers have evaluated the effectiveness of Stem Cell Therapy and tissue engineering for treating osteoarthritis. Both bone marrow and adipose-derived stem cells have the potential to provide a permanent biological solution. Although one study suggests that there are more stem cells in adipose than in bone marrow, it is not clear whether the number of cells is important, since stem cells divide logarithmically inside the body.

The studies cited below found that bone marrow stem cells are more effective than adipose stem cells.

From researchers at the Institutes of Immunology and Pathology, Rikshospitalet University Hospital in Norway: "We have compared articular chondrocytes with MSC from human bone marrow (BM) and adipose tissue (AT), all cultured in HA scaffolds, for their ability to express genes and synthesize proteins associated with chondrogenesis. The cells were expanded in monolayer cultures. The results were that Chondrogenesis in HA scaffolds was more efficient using BM-MSC than AT-MSC or chondrocytes."[14]

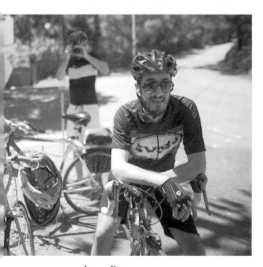

Jason Darrow

From researchers at the Stem Cell Biology Department, Stem Cell Technology Research Center, Tehran, Iran: "BM-MSC showed the highest capacity for osteogenic differentiation and hold promising potential for bone tissue engineering and cell therapy applications compared to AD-MSC. The growth factor genes were expressed more in the differentiated state in BMC compared to adipose tissue."[15]

A greater improvement was seen with bone marrow-derived mesenchymal stem cells when compared to adipose-derived stromal vascular fraction and placebo treatment in this horse clinical study from researchers at Colorado State University.[16]

This study from the Department of Orthopaedics at the Affiliated Hospital of Guilin Medical College, Guilin, China, demonstrated bone-marrow-MSCs to have greater in-vivo chondrogenic potential than periosteum, synovium, adipose, and muscle MSCs.[17]

In a large animal model from Freiburg University Hospital in Germany, ASC seem to be inferior to BMSC in terms of osteogenic potential, but that can partially be compensated by the addition of PRP to the ASC. However, BMSC already has PRP within the solution, so no PRP needs to be added to this group.[18]

In this horse model from Louisiana State University, equine BMSCs have superior chondrogenic potential compared with ASCs.[19]

Doctors in Taiwan noted that: Mesenchymal stem cells (MSCs) isolated from either bone marrow or adipose tissue show considerable promise for use in cartilage repair. The MSCs can be sourced from any or all joint tissues and can modulate the immune response. Additionally, MSCs can directly differentiate into chondrocytes under appropriate signal transduction. They also have immunosuppressive and anti-inflammatory paracrine effects. (They change the joint environment from breakdown to healing by telling the other cells to start repairing.)[20]

An Interesting Observation from Surgeons

In an editorial in the January 2016 issue of the *Journal of Arthroscopic and Related Surgery*, Associate Editor Merrick J. Wetzler, M.D., wrote: "Harvesting of the ADSCs [fat stem cells] does require an additional procedure, and the cost-effectiveness of the procedure is still under investigation, but as researchers stated in their editorials in 2012 and 2013, 'We are believers in Stem Cell Therapy' and 'Stem cells have substantial potential to allow 21st century physicians and surgeons . . . to achieve unprecedented tissue healing and repair.'

"We do believe that it is only a matter of time before the harvesting and growth of stem cells will become cost-effective and commercially available and will be added to our treatment options for restoration of articular cartilage."

That is a good endorsement from surgeons—however, as Dr. Wetzler noted, there is an added cost of the stem cell procedure using adipose (fat) stem cells, along with the more complex harvesting procedure involved in obtaining the fat cells.

Nevertheless, there is more research pending on the value of stem cells from bone marrow vs fat, and other doctors in the field have not concurred on the best modality. In time, studies will most likely provide the answer. And since the field is fairly new, much more exploration is required.

Beyond Osteoarthritis—Treatment of Tendinopathies

Are bone marrow stem cells the new player in nonsurgical tendon repair? In the latest research, doctors writing in the medical journal

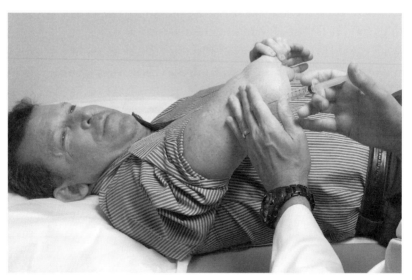

Randy Weinzoff, DC

Hand Surgery suggest that bone-marrow derived stem cells accelerate tendon healing in animal studies.[21]

Doctors know that chronic tendon injuries present unique management challenges because of the long-held belief that they result from ongoing inflammation. This thinking has caused physicians to rely on treatments demonstrated to be ineffective in the long term— e.g., anti-inflammatory medications and cortisone shots.

This is why there is mounting excitement about Stem Cell Therapy. Published in the *Journal of Muscles Ligaments Tendons*, researchers from Italy wrote: "Tendon injuries represent, even today, a challenge, as repair may be exceedingly slow and incomplete. Regenerative medicine and stem cell technology have shown to be of great promise."[22]

Most recently, a study from the Feinstein Institute for Medical Research indicated the potential effectiveness of bone marrow (stem cells) for Achilles tendon healing, particularly during the early phases.[23]

Am I Too Old for Stem Cell Therapy?

A recent study from the journal *American Health and Drug Benefits* suggests that to save on national health care costs, patients over the age of 70 should just have a knee replacement and not even explore steroid or hyaluronic acid (viscosupplementation injections).[24]

In recent research, doctors have noted that health care interventions for knee osteoarthritis are poorly perceived, and that patients expect the "inevitable" joint replacement. The expected failure of conservative treatment to manage pain and symptoms is common partly because clinicians frequently trivialize osteoarthritis.[25]

This is almost paradoxical. The patients are too old for other treatments, yet some doctors suggest that they should simply proceed to the most invasive and dangerous treatment that requires the most healing and recovery time. What is too old for a knee replacement? And, what is too old for extended recovery and rehabilitation? Evidently, there is no limit.

In another recent study in the medical journal *Transplantation*, researchers reported results of Stem Cell Therapy in patients who showed rapid and progressive improvement (in function), with enhanced knee cartilage quality. "[Stem Cell Therapy] . . . may be a valid alternative treatment for chronic knee osteoarthritis. The intervention is simple, does not require hospitalization or surgery, provides pain relief, and significantly improves cartilage quality."[26]

National University of Ireland researchers suggest that stem cells should be considered as reservoirs of repair cells that fix damaged joint tissue, strengthen the healthy joint tissue while also repairing the problems associated with chronic inflammation (swelling and stiffness).[27] Duke University research agrees and adds that stem cells are viable even in elderly patients who may yet still display significant chondrogenic (cartilage regrowth) potential.[28]

In the hands of an experienced practitioner who is familiar with joint injections and the healing properties of Stem Cell Therapy, this treatment can be ideal for repairing and regenerating joint cartilage. I invite you to continue reading this book to see how stem cells can help you avoid unnecessary and dangerous joint replacement, elective orthopedic surgery, or spinal surgery.

3

Platelet-Rich Plasma Therapy (PRP)

As stated in Chapter 1, "Chronic complex musculo-skeletal injuries that are slow to heal pose challenges to physicians and researchers alike. Orthobiologics is a relatively new science that involves application of naturally found materials from biological sources (blood platelets and stem cells among them), and offers exciting new possibilities to promote and accelerate bone and soft tissue healing.

"Platelet-rich plasma (PRP) is an orthobiologic that has recently gained popularity as an adjuvant treatment for musculoskeletal injuries. It is a volume of fractionated plasma from the patient's own blood that contains platelet concentrate. The platelets contain alpha granules that are rich in several growth factors which play key roles in tissue repair mechanisms. PRP has found application in diverse surgical fields to enhance bone and soft tissue healing by placing supra-physiological concentrations of autologous platelets at the site of tissue damage. The

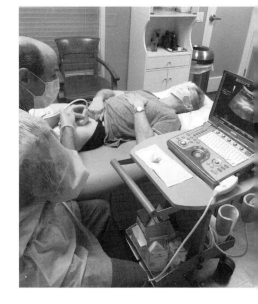

relative ease of prepara-
tion, applicability in the
clinical setting, favorable
safety profile and possible
beneficial outcome make
PRP a promising thera-
peutic approach for future
regenerative treatments." [29]

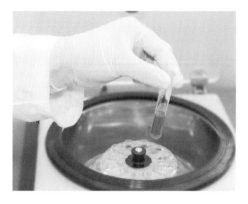

The above was written
in 2012 from researchers
at the University of Rochester to support the adjuvant use (i.e., aiding healing after the surgery) of PRP. Since that research was done,
numerous medical studies have suggested that PRP has found favor
with surgeons for helping heal postsurgical damage. Other researchers
have demonstrated benefits of the simpler injection treatment of PRP
to help patients avoid surgery.

How Does PRP Therapy Work?

PRP treatments involve collecting a small amount of your blood and
spinning it in a centrifuge to separate the platelets from the red cells.
The collected platelets are then injected back into the injured area
to stimulate healing and regeneration. PRP puts specific components
in the blood to work. Blood is made up of four main components;
plasma, red blood cells, white blood cells, and platelets. Each part
plays a role in keeping your body functioning properly. Platelets act
as wound and injury healers. They are first on the scene at an injury,
clotting to stop any bleeding and immediately helping to regenerate
new tissue in the wounded area.

The platelets contain healing agents or "growth factors." Let's look
at some of the growth factors and what they do:

- Platelet-derived growth factor (PDGF) is a protein that helps control cell growth and division, especially blood vessels. When more
blood (and the oxygen it carries) is delivered to the site of a wound,
there is more healing.

- Transforming growth factor beta (or TGF-β) is a polypeptide and is important in tissue regeneration.
- Insulin-like growth factors are signaling agents. They help change the environment of the damaged joint from diseased to healing by "signaling" the immune system to start rebuilding tissue.
- Vascular endothelial growth factor (VEGF) is an important protein that brings healing oxygen to damaged tissue where blood circulation might be damaged or inadequate.
- Epidermal growth factor plays a key role in tissue repair mechanisms.

We discuss the use of platelet-rich plasma (PRP) throughout this book. In this introductory chapter we focus on PRP's broad application as supported in the medical literature.

PRP for Bone Healing and Regeneration

Researchers at the University of Memphis and Saint Louis University acknowledge that there is little doubt that the growth factor milieu contained within PRP has the potential to be highly beneficial to bone regeneration.[30]

In fact, PRP is such a promising treatment for bone regeneration that doctors also support the use of PRP for large bone defects to assist healing and bone regeneration.[31] Researchers have confirmed that PRP accelerates the healing and growth of bone in large-bone tumor-created defects and other defects.[32, 33] It is also being studied for routine use in regeneration of cystic bony defects (characteristics of bone tumors) in children.[34]

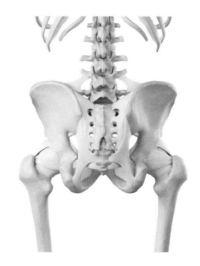

Hip Osteoarthritis

Researchers at the University of Florence found that the majority of patients receiving PRP for hip osteoarthritis had significant pain reduction at 6-7 weeks that was sustained at 6 months, and they also had better range of motion.[35]

More Italian research from the Rizzoli Orthopedic Institute showed improved findings: "Results indicated that intra-articular PRP injections offer a significant clinical improvement in patients with hip osteoarthritis without relevant side effects."[36]

Even after hip surgery, researchers in Chile noted that PRP was effective in reducing pain that continued after the surgery.[37]

Hip OA is treated almost daily in my office. The most amazing recovery is that of a man who was a life-long body builder. His left hip was almost fused, with no range of motion. I refused to treat the hip since I didn't think PRP would help. Instead I used PRP on his right knee. After some success with his knee he begged me to inject his hip. I finally did, and to my surprise, he was then able to reach down to the floor to pick up weights. A movement he could not do for years before.

Degenerative Disc Disease

Research has shown PRP to be effective in treating degenerative disc disease (DDD) by addressing the problems of spinal ligament instability and by stimulating the regeneration of the discs indirectly (although discs were not directly injected, they showed an increase in disc height).[38]

Research presented by international scientists in Milan in August 2015 showed that PRP is able to recover the mechanical properties of denatured (worn-down) discs, thereby providing a promising effective therapeutic modality.[39]

Although I don't typically consider DDD to be a major player in neck or back pain, I do treat these areas daily. From my exam, it is typically not the discs that are the issue, but the ligaments at their connection to bone that cause the pain. This is called an enthesopathy. And typically, it is easy to heal with PRP. Please be very careful to not have surgery for areas that can heal with PRP. As you will read, areas in MRIs that show anatomical issues, may not be the pain generator.

Knee Osteoarthritis (OA)

One study showed that "[I]ntra-knee articular injection of PRP to treat knee articular cartilage degeneration is safe, [and] can alleviate symptoms of pain and swelling and improve the quality of life of patients."[40] Researchers in Barcelona, Spain were able to report results at six months which showed improvements in patients' knee function and quality of life.[41]

Another study from doctors in Thailand found that PRP produced greater improvement in knees than hyaluronic acid injection and placebos in terms of reducing symptoms and improving function, as well as in improving quality of life.[42] In a study from the Mayo Clinic, PRP was seen to be more effective than hyaluronic acid in younger, active patients with low-grade osteoarthritis.[43]

PRP has demonstrated significant improvements in *Knee Injury and Osteoarthritis Outcome Scores*, including pain and symptom relief, in addition to having the ability to provide pain relief, halt progression of meniscal damage, and regenerate tissue.[44, 45]

In supportive research in the surgical journal *Arthroscopy*, doctors concluded that PRP injections are a viable treatment for knee osteoarthritis and should be considered for patients with this condition.[46]

Studies like these add to the accumulating evidence that PRP can halt and reverse meniscus degeneration.[47, 48, 49]

The most common issue that I see in the office is knee OA. I inject PRP and stem cells into many knees every day. I use an ultrasound to guide the needle to make sure the solution enters the joint. Without ultrasound guidance, there is a 33% chance that the solution will actually miss the joint, and end up in the soft tissue. Not only will that not be a healing action, but it can cause a huge inflammatory reaction with an effusion (fluid in the knee). I have heard patients say that having a baby was easier.

Kneecap and Tendons

Patellar tendinopathy, often called "runner's knee," is a condition that has been shown to respond very favorably to Platelet-Rich Plasma

Therapy. Researchers in the Netherlands reported: "After PRP treatment, patients with patellar tendinopathy showed a statistically significant and meaningful improvement."[50]

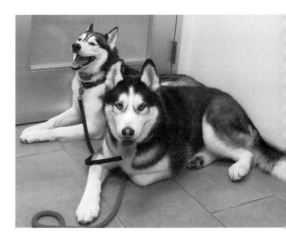

My 80 pound Husky, Dakota, was running with me at the dog park. I let him take off, and I only saw him for a second prior to him hitting me full speed on the lateral side of my left knee. Although the blow was to the lateral or outside of the knee, I felt the pain on the medial or inside of the knee. I actually felt the joint open up, and remembered "O'Donaghue's terrible triad." I couldn't believe this happened to me. It was common years ago when football players wanted to "take out" a player, and they would roll onto the side of a player's knee. The result can be ACL, medial meniscus, and medial collateral ligament tears, all at one time. In addition, my patella loosened and started to catch in the trochlear groove of the femur when I flexed or extended my knee. Running was painful, and my two-miler in the hills with my Huskies each morning was becoming more and more painful. Injecting patients, and bracing my knee on the table became painful, and the clicking became worse. I injected my knee ten times with dextrose (old style Prolotherapy) over a 3 month period, and each time the knee would improve a bit, but running would loosen it again. I finally had my staff draw my blood, and injected the joint, and about twenty other areas around the patella. Within minutes, the knee tightened up, and the crepitus (clicking) stopped. By the time I got home, my knee was stiff, but certainly tolerable. It remained stiff till about 11 am the next morning, and then felt normal again. To allow enough tissue to grow, I withheld running for 2 weeks, even though I felt good the next day. When I did run, the Huskies pulled me at full speed, and my knee was as good as new. I had another minor injury to my knee many months later from over indulging in "posting" on my left knee during endless hours of golf practice. I reinjected myself with PRP, and 5 days later, ran full speed with the Huskies, pulling hard. Again, I ran pain free, and no thought of an injury. I always tell my patients to wait much longer to exercise an area that I inject, but for me, I can reinject any time I like for free.

Rotator Cuff—Shoulder

Injections of PRP have led to reduced pain and improved recovery for the treatment of rotator cuff tears.[51, 52] PRP also enhances rotator cuff repair following arthroscopic shoulder surgery.[53]

At a meeting of the American Academy of Orthopaedic Surgeons, researchers suggested that PRP injections may be a safe and cost-effective treatment alternative for rotator cuff tendinopathy (RCT).[54]

My experience is that it also works on full-thickness tears. I inject shoulders every day, and have seen patients who can't lift their arm because of a tear, get pain free, complete range of motion.

Doctors in Switzerland compared PRP injections to cortisone injections and concluded that PRP injections are a good alternative, especially in patients with contraindications to cortisone.[52] To me all patients have contraindications to cortisone since it thins the tissue and can be a set-up for injury.

Normal   **Rotator cuff problems**

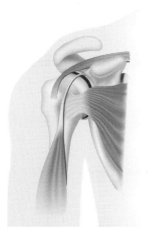 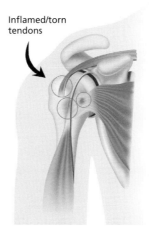

Inflamed/torn tendons

Tennis Elbow

Patients with chronic lateral epicondylitis, known as tennis elbow, received PRP injections once or twice at four-week intervals in a recent study, complemented with standardized physical therapy. Six months after the localized PRP treatment, these patients reported significant pain relief and gain in function, as well as improved quality of life. Accoring to doctors at the Rizzoli Orthopedic Institute and University of Bologna in Italy, a single PRP injection may be sufficient.[55] Doctors from the United Kingdom confirmed these findings, showing that PRP injections have an important and effective role in treatment of the elbow, especially in difficult cases of tennis elbow.[56]

As with all parts of the body, I inject elbows on an almost daily basis. For a reason, unknown to me, even when the problem appears to be on the outside tendon of the elbow, an additional PRP injecton into the joint seems to speed healing.

Achilles Tendinopathies—Ankle/Foot

For patients with Achilles tendinopathy and plantar fasciitis, PRP was found to be an effective and safe alternative for those with a poor response to conventional nonsurgical treatments in two studies.[57, 58]

In a of study patients affected by mid-portion Chronic Recalcitrant Achilles Tendinopathies, PRP was found to be effective even in a single treatment.[59] Again, these are areas common to my injections. Ultrasound is a necessity to guide a needle to the plantar fascia attachment on the calcaneus (heel bone). The common approach is through the bottom of the foot which is very painful, but with an ultrasound, the needle can be guided through the less sensitive medial surface of the foot.

TMJ-Osteoarthritis—Jaw

Doctors in Egypt studied 50 patients with TMJ-osteoarthritis. They found that PRP performed better than hyaluronic acid during long-term follow-up in terms of pain reduction and increased interincisal distance—that is, the ability to open one's mouth wider.[60] In a study done in Turkey, researchers concluded that patients suffering from temporomandibular joint (TMJ) disc dislocation benefited more from PRP injections than from surgery to manipulate the jaw back into place. Clearly, PRP stabilized the joint and reduced chronic instability.[61]

One of my patients was in a terrible bus accident which included death and amputation of two of his relatives. His jaw was fractured as a result of the accident. His mouth had been wired shut for three months and he had minimal range of motion of the jaw for months thereafter. After a few treatments of PRP, he had full range of jaw motion, and was able reach his goal of eating a Big Mac.

I have had several other patients ready for TMJ surgery, who after a few treatments were pain free with full range of motion.

A study in Poland found that platelet-rich plasma injections into the temporomandibular joint had a positive impact on the reduction of the intensity of pain experienced by patients who were being treated for TMJ dysfunction.[62]

PRP is Safe and Effective

The use of platelet-rich plasma for chronic joint pain holds great promise. As more research comes in, it is increasingly clear that PRP is effective for the treatment of chronic pain caused by injury or by "wear-and-tear" arthritis.

There are minimal risks associated with PRP treatment. In fact, doctors found that PRP helped patients who had other medical conditions that can make healing more difficult, such as diabetes and heart disease.[63]

As an old-style Prolotherapist, I have injected most parts of the body, literally from head to toe. What I have found is that PRP works substantially better than the old-style dextrose injections of Prolotherapy, and stem cells work substantially better than PRP. This will be discussed later.

PART TWO

Treating Specific Conditions

4

Knee Pain

It used to be that if a doctor told you, "I'm recommending arthroscopic surgery to clean up your knee" or "You need a total knee replacement," you had just two choices: surgery or painkillers.

With the advent of "biomedicine" (blood and stem cell therapies and injections), the choices have changed dramatically. From this point of view, arthroscopic surgery is now seen as the least desirable option, and knee replacement something that should be delayed as long as possible. Stimulating the growth of cartilage and damaged or worn tissue is now seen as the most desirable option.

In 2015, studies on Stem Cell Therapy and knee cartilage began to be published at an amazing rate.

The reason for this explosion in research is simple: doctors and patients are seeing poor results from surgery, along with unexpected side effects, and the powerful new tools of biomedicine are thus becoming a major focus.

Here is the introduction to one study from a combined team of European researchers:

"The therapeutic potential of mesenchymal stromal cells (MSCs, or stem cells) is evident by the number of new and ongoing trials targeting an impressive variety of conditions.

"In bone and cartilage repair, MSCs are expected to replace the damaged tissue, while in other therapies they modulate a therapeutic response by the secretion of bioactive molecules. [That is, they rally the stem cells already in the damaged joint through chemical messaging to get to work repairing damage.]

MSCs possess a phenotypic plasticity [they can change into other cells] and harbor an arsenal of bioactive molecules [healing cells] that can be released upon sensing signals."[64]

Before biomedicine, stem cells, and blood platelets, the gold standard of treatment for patients suffering from debilitating joint pain due to a "bone-on-bone" condition was joint replacement. However, as the decades progressed, patients who had received replacement therapy grew older, and their prosthetic joints began to wear out.

Doctors became aware of a new challenge for themselves and their patients, one that did not have an easy solution. In older joint replacements, bone was removed and replaced with metal. When a revision (second) replacement was needed, some patients no longer had enough bone to have this surgery.

These patients' knees, shoulders, and hips became "salvage" jobs, as doctors tried to do what they could with whatever was left of the original joint. During my internship, after a patient's surgical hip joint replacement failure, I assisted my mentor in carving an entire femur from a cadaver, and placing it into the pelvis and knee to create new joints. The chance for success was minimal, but at least amputation was postponed—for good or bad, I am not sure.

Problems with Knee Replacement

While knee replacement can sometimes be a viable and effective treatment for patients with knee osteoarthritis, the number of patients asking about knee replacement alternatives continues to grow. Patients need to be aware of the potential downsides of the procedure, particularly in light of the new therapies available.

In the *British Medical Journal*, investigators examined why 10–34% of patients who had had a knee replacement still had knee pain. What they found was that there was no matrix to predict whether or not a knee replacement surgery would be successful. In fact, doctors were asked to devise a plan that was lacking: "Our systematic review highlights the lack of evidence about prediction and management of chronic postsurgical pain after total knee replacement. Given the complexity of chronic postsurgical pain and the range of possible treatment options, screening and adequate referral processes are needed, so that patients can receive appropriate interventions that have the potential to improve outcomes and reduce distress. As a large number of people are affected by chronic pain after total knee replacement, the development of an evidence base about care for these patients should be a research priority."[65]

Over the years I have seen many patients who still had knee pain following knee replacement surgery. What I see in my practice agrees with what medical research states—that knee replacement surgery offers hope to some patients, and these patients have high expectations of what the new knee will offer them, but that in many cases those expectations are not met.

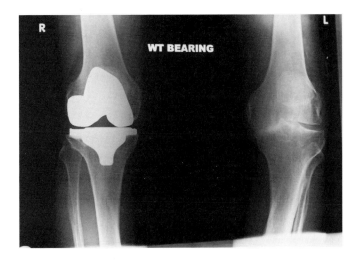

Patients are catching on. In a recent medical survey, patients who were given educational materials about knee replacement and more time to decide, ultimately decided to at least postpone the surgery.[66]

Providing information to patients is important. In one study of patients who had had knee replacements, researchers reported: "Despite high expectations, there were statistically and clinically significant differences between actual and expected activity at 12 months, suggesting that expectations may not have been fulfilled."[67]

In other words, the researchers found that the patients could not perform activities as they had hoped following knee replacement.

This is what a new study from doctors at the New York Hospital for Special Surgery says: "Although total knee replacement is a successful and cost-effective procedure, patient dissatisfaction remains as high as 50%."[68]

Recently, in more startling research, doctors said that too many people were getting knee replacements, and that up to one-third of them really did not need the procedure.

Here is material from a press release issued by *Arthritis & Rheumatology*, a journal of the American College of Rheumatology:

> "The Agency for Healthcare Research and Quality reports more than 600,000 knee replacements are performed in the U.S. each year. In the past 15 years, the use of total knee arthroplasty has grown significantly, with studies showing an annual volume increase of 162% in Medicare-covered knee replacement surgeries between 1991 and 2010. Some experts believe the growth is due to the use of an effective procedure, while others contend there is overuse of the surgery that relies on subjective criteria.
>
> A study led by Dr. Daniel Riddle of the Department of Physical Therapy at Virginia Commonwealth University in Richmond, Va., examined the criteria used to determine the appropriateness of total knee arthroplasties. Dr. Riddle concluded, "Analyses show that 44% of surgeries were classified as appropriate, 22% as inconclusive, and 34% [were] deemed inappropriate." [69, 70]

Reasons for Knee Replacement Failure

The presentation of knee instability can vary from pain to dislocation, with the origins of the pain varied and sometimes undetermined. Instability after total knee replacement can also be classified by where it occurs in the knee's arc of motion.

Acute instability is related to intraoperative injuries or excessive release of important coronal stabilizers, such as the medial collateral ligament in extension or the posterolateral corner in flexion (bending).

Chronic instability in extension is often related to varus/valgus malalignment (i.e., the replacement knee was installed incorrectly).[71]

Finally, knee replacements sometimes fail because the patient's back or hip pain was mistaken for knee pain. [72]

PAINKILLERS AND OPIOIDS DO NOT WORK

Doctors at Stanford published their findings on the problems of painkillers: "Patients taking opioids (narcotic painkillers) prior to surgery experience prolonged postoperative opioid use, worsened clinical outcomes, increased pain, and gave more postoperative complications."[73]

If you have been taking painkillers for a long time and then have a knee replacement, you will have a higher risk of more pain and complication following the surgery, because painkillers inhibit healing.

In a report in the *American Journal of Bone and Joint Surgery*, Canadian researchers came to the same conclusion:

"Chronic use of opioid medications may lead to dependence or hyperalgesia, both of which might adversely affect perioperative and postoperative pain management, rehabilitation, and clinical outcomes after total knee arthroplasty. The purpose of this study was to evaluate patients who underwent total knee arthroplasty following six or more weeks of chronic opioid use for pain control and to compare them with a matched group who did not use opioids preoperatively.

"A significantly higher prevalence of complications was seen in the opioid group, with five arthroscopic evaluations and eight revisions for persistent stiffness and/or pain, compared with none in the matched group. Ten patients in the opioid group were referred for outpatient pain management, compared with one patient in the non-opioid group.

"Conclusions: Patients who chronically use opioid medications prior to total knee arthroplasty may be at a substantially greater risk for complications and painful prolonged recoveries. Alternative non-opioid pain medications and/or earlier referral to an orthopaedic surgeon prior to habitual opioid use should be considered for patients with painful degenerative disease of the knee."[74]

PSYCHOLOGICAL FACTORS

Despite the development of multimodal analgesia for postoperative pain management, doctors say opioids are still required for effective pain relief after knee replacement.[75]

Doctors at the Icahn School of Medicine at Mount Sinai Hopsital in New York gave their opinion in research from 2016: "Total knee replacement is associated with substantial postoperative pain that may impair mobility, reduce the ability to participate in rehabilitation, lead to chronic pain, and reduce patient satisfaction. Traditional general anesthesia with postoperative epidural and patient-controlled opioid analgesia is associated with an undesirable adverse-effect profile, including postoperative nausea and vomiting, hypotension, urinary retention, respiratory depression, delirium, and an increased infection rate."[76]

Realistic goals in knee replacement must be discussed with patients who think knee replacement will ease their depression or anxiety about health and other concerns.

Doctors at the University of Nottingham in the UK announced in their findings: "Approximately 10–25% of patients are reportedly dissatisfied with the results of bicondylar knee prosthesis implantation. Psychopathologic factors, particularly somatization dysfunction [anxiety], have an impact on total knee replacement outcomes.

Preoperative screening and concurrent treatment of the diagnosed psychological disorder may improve patient-perceived outcomes."[77]

From a study at the Martin Luther teaching hospital in Germany: "Knee replacement surgery reduces pain for many people with osteoarthritis. However, surgical outcomes are partly dependent on patients' moods, and those with depression or anxiety have worse outcomes. Approximately one-third of people with osteoarthritis have mood problems according to research.[78]

This from research lead by doctors at the University of Turin: "A significant number of patients in this [study] undergoing routine primary total knee replacement had signs of subclinical depression. These patients are more likely to report increased pain even at one year following surgery compared to patients without signs of depression preoperatively. Psychometric evaluation prior to surgery can help identify the at-risk patient and allow for proper management of patient expectations."[79]

A study from Monash University "found evidence for a relationship between cognitive factors, but not behavioural factors, and knee pain. Coping, self-efficacy, somatising (anxiety), pain catastrophizing and helplessness were grouped together as 'cognitive factors,' while kinesiophobia [the fear of movement] and pain-related fear avoidance were considered 'behavioural' factors."[80]

Others researching the connection between emotions and knee pain reported: "Psychological functioning plays an important role in knee pain, with strong evidence for depression being associated with knee pain . . . . This is important given the increasing understanding of the complexity of knee pain and potential complications arising from many of the treatments in current use. A holistic approach to managing knee pain has the potential to improve patient outcomes."[81]

PHYSICAL LIMITATIONS FOLLOWING KNEE REPLACEMENT

New and concerning research is out about how quickly someone getting a total knee replacement is able to return to work.

The research says that an increasing number of patients in the working population are undergoing total knee replacement for end-stage osteoarthritis. The timing and success of their return to work is becoming increasingly important for this group of patients, with social and economic implications for patients and their employers.

The concern is that patients have a limited understanding of the realistic variables that determine the ability to return to work. In other words—they think they can get back to work sooner than they will actually be able to.

In speaking with knee-replacement patients, the researchers found that the patients had a great deal of concern, primarily involving these three factors:

1. The time delay in getting the surgery (i.e., being on a long waiting list)
2. Limited and often inconsistent advice from health care professionals regarding when they would be able to return to work
3. The absence of rehabilitation that would optimize recovery and facilitate the return to work

The patients felt that all of these factors contributed to potential delays in a successful return to work.[82]

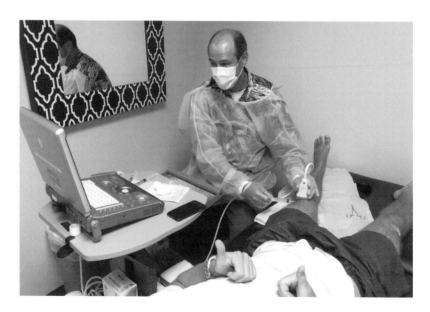

Stem Cells Instead of Knee Replacement

It became clear to many researchers that joint replacement had to be redefined and disputed as the gold standard of treatment. Others, however, had already decided to abandon joint replacement and explore growing tissue as the new standard of care. The thinking was simple—why remove bone and tissue when these could be repaired and rejuvenated?

What was found in the initial research was startling. Doctors discovered that one type of stem cell (mesenchymal stem cells found in bone marrow and body fat) could morph into bone cells and cartilage cells when injected into a joint. The ramifications for the treatment of osteoarthritis or "bone-on-bone" joints were enormous. Stem cell injections showed that cartilage could be regrown, something that doctors had previously thought impossible because of the cartilage's limited blood supply within the joint. Most recently, doctors announced that they had confirmed successful regeneration of cartilage tissue in the knee through simple Stem Cell Therapy injection.[83, 84]

Research on the Effectiveness of Platelet-Rich Plasma Therapy (PRP) for Knee Osteoarthritis

Recently, numerous studies have appeared on the effectiveness of PRP in treating knee osteoarthritis.

In one study, doctors found that in a follow-up done after a year or less, patients receiving PRP injections had improved functional outcomes when compared to patients who had received either hyaluronic acid or placebo.[85] PRP seems to be more effective than hyaluronic acid in younger, active patients with low-grade osteoarthritis.[86] In the medical journal *International Orthopaedics*, researchers showed that PRP enhances and accelerates the healing process.[87]

Research like that above help doctors conclude: "(PRP injections) to treat knee articular cartilage degeneration is safe . . . can alleviate symptoms of pain and swelling and improve the quality of life of patients."[88]

Surgery to Repair Damaged Cartilage in the Knee

Doctors are trying to identify which surgery works best for cartilage damage in the knee. However, in one research paper in the journal *Sports Health*, doctors acknowledge that deciding which surgery works best is a difficult clinical challenge, particularly in younger patients, for whom alternatives such as partial or total knee arthroplasty are rarely advised.

These doctors noted numerous surgical techniques that have been developed to address cartilage defects and are characterized as follows:

- Palliation (e.g., chondroplasty, which is surgery to smooth out cartilage) and debridement (power washing of the knee cartilage)
- Repair (e.g., drilling and microfracture [MFI])
- Tansplant restoration (e.g., autologous chondrocyte implantation [ACI], osteochondral autograft [OAT], and osteochondral allograft [OCA])

In the study the authors concluded: "These techniques may improve patient outcomes, though no single technique can reproduce normal hyaline cartilage."[89]

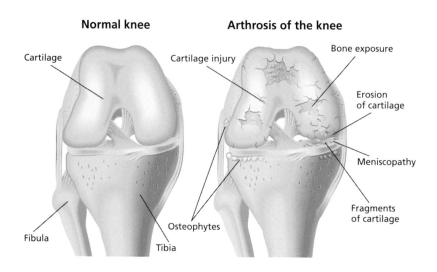

Normal knee

Cartilage

Fibula

Tibia

Arthrosis of the knee

Cartilage injury

Bone exposure

Erosion of cartilage

Meniscopathy

Fragments of cartilage

Osteophytes

In agreement are Ohio State University researchers who say: "The markedly limited healing potential of articular cartilage often leads these patients to continued deterioration and progressive functional limitations even after surgery."[90]

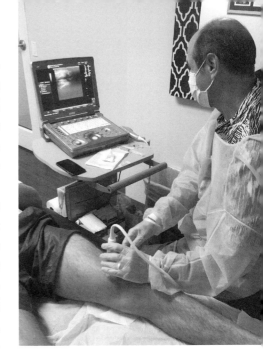

However, some of the procedures did get younger athletes back to their sport. Athletes are allowed to return to sports participation after autologous chondrocyte implantation, osteochondral autograft, or osteochondral allograft (donor cadaver cartilage), and microfracture, although microfracture patients are the least likely to return to sports.

Patients with the best prognosis after surgery had the following characteristics:

- younger
- shorter preoperative duration of symptoms
- no previous surgical interventions
- participated in a more rigorous rehabilitation protocol
- had smaller cartilage defects[91]

Most of the patients I see in my practice have a history of surgical procedures, lengthy duration of symptoms, and a history of multiple and varied treatments. As researchers note, the markedly limited healing potential of articular cartilage often leads such patients toward continued deterioration and progressive functional limitations.[92]

Platelet-Rich Plasma Therapy (PRP) for Osteochondral Defect

The problem with surgery is that it cannot do what most athletes want most, which is to repair and regrow damaged tissue quickly so they can get back to their sport. No single surgery will regrow cartilage—something that Stem Cell Therapy and PRP *can* do.

Surgeons did find that PRP and Stem Cell Therapy assisted healing:

"Advances in the understanding of tissue repair mechanisms and the pivotal role of growth factors have stimulated the use of platelet-rich therapies by orthopaedic surgeons and sports physicians, mainly with the aim of stimulating and enhancing tissue healing."[93]

This would seem like the best of both worlds—surgery employing a healing agent that regrows cartilage. The question is: Why would they use these cells during surgery when they could be used by themselves, *without* an invasive surgical procedure? And, why cut tissue out, only to try to grow it back?

Further, many studies have found that PRP and surgery do not work well together.[94] This is possibly due to the damage created by the surgery itself.

Recent research warns doctors against using injectables following arthroscopic surgery, because the arthroscopic fluids greatly dilute the benefits of solutions. If ever there were a double-edged sword, this is it—the surgery causes damage, and the surgical fluids dilute the beneficial healing factors.

Knee Cartilage Transplant (Autologous Chondrocyte Implantation)

Writing in the *American Journal of Sports Medicine*, doctors had this to say: In the face of the fact that there are no effective drugs or surgery capable of restoring the original structure and function of damaged articular cartilage, researchers have focused on alternatives such as biological therapies for osteoarthritis and related orthopaedic disorders. One such alternative is autologous chondrocyte implantation (ACI).

Long considered by many to be the "go-to" procedure for treatment of osteoarticular damage and tears, ACI has been used for over two decades. Prior to scheduling surgery, a piece of healthy cartilage is first taken from an area that does not further compromise the knee. From this cartilage, chondrocytes—the specialized cells that create the cartilage—are separated and cultured. Over the next few weeks, if enough cells are grown, a surgery is scheduled in which the chondrocytes are implanted into the defective cartilage.

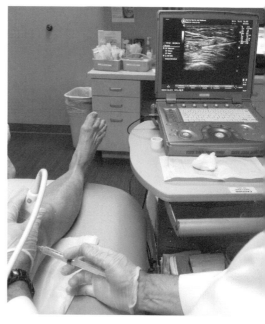

Although chondrocyte-based therapy (cartilage transplantation) has the capacity to slow the progression of osteoarthritis and delay partial or total joint replacement surgery, currently used procedures are associated with the risk of serious adverse events.

Autologous Chondrocyte Transplantation has the disadvantage of requiring two surgical interventions as well as the in-vitro expansion of cells, implying the risk of cellular de-differentiation (i.e., the transplant does not hold). Further, for those who perform high-level activities—such as sports or physically demanding work—the patch is not seen as reliable.[95]

Stem Cells for Repairing Cartilage

Obviously, for surgeons there is a significant interest in improving the success rate of ACI by improving surgical techniques and preserving the natural state of the implanted cells.[96]

Stem cells are considered an answer. By bringing Stem Cell Therapy into the surgery, doctors feel that their cartilage transplants will work better. The question here is this: If stem cells will make the surgery more successful, why not try Stem Cell Therapy first, before going to surgery? After all, stem cell injections on their own have shown remarkable results in research and at my clinic—and without the serious complications of the ACI procedure.

In animal studies, researchers note: "Mesenchymal stem cells (MSCs) represent a promising alternative form of cell-based therapy for cartilage injury." In a comparison study, Stem Cell Therapy was found to do the same, even for full-thickness tears. The results have an implication of supporting the potential use of stem cells for cartilage repair in cases of sports injuries or disease, offering similar efficacy but reduced patient risk and potential cost savings compared with conventional Autologous Chondrocyte Implantation therapy.[97]

Hyaluronic Acid

Doctors are suggesting that if you want more hyaluronic acid in your knees, Stem Cell Therapy may be an answer.

Investigators examined the interaction of bone marrow-derived mesenchymal stem cells and osteoarthritic cartilage cells in the production of natural hyaluronan (hyaluronic acid) in the knee. Their results indicated that when bone marrow-derived stem cells are introduced into an arthritic joint, they change their behavior and the healing environment by increasing production of hyaluronan or "hyaluronic acid."[98]

Frequently, my new patients state that they have reached their "allowable limit of hyaluronic acid injections" and that their doctor is prescribing surgery. Their question is whether Stem Cell Therapy or Platelet-Rich Plasma Therapy (PRP) can help save them from surgery.

Recently doctors warned that "while hyaluronic acid injections can provide significant pain relief and improvement in the knee, this may cause excessive loading on the knee joints, which may further accelerate the rate of knee degeneration." Do hyaluronic acid injections cause knee degeneration? The answer is yes, because hyaluronic acid does not regenerate tissue.[99]

Another study suggests that PRP injections are more effective than hyaluronic acid injections in reducing symptoms and improving quality of life.[100] And a recent randomized controlled trial in Spain found

PRP therapy to be superior to hyaluronic acid injections in alleviating symptoms of mild to moderate osteoarthritis of the knee.[101]

While doctors are saying that hyaluronic acid injections may be effective in pain reduction, there is no data supporting the regeneration of cartilage and meniscus tissue.[102] However, PRP *can* regenerate this tissue, which is why the investigators suggested that it was a superior treatment.[103]

While the above research suggests that PRP should be chosen over hyaluronic acid injections, researchers writing in the French medical journal *Prescrire international* suggest that intra-articular hyaluronic acid injections for osteoarthritis of the knee should be avoided completely: "At best, intra-articular hyaluronic acid injections give modest relief to patients suffering knee osteoarthritis pain, at the price of local reactions and sometimes severe adverse effects."[104]

I have seen patients require incision and drainage with antibiotic treatment after experiencing allergic reactions to hyaluronic acid injections. When the injections are mistakenly placed into the soft tissue instead of the joint, severe reactions can occur. Studies have confirmed that when knee injections are made blindly—that is, without ultrasound guidance—one-third of the injections do not enter the joint. Unfortunately, most doctors do not inject under ultrasound guidance.

MRIs—Useful or Useless for Knee Pain?

I often receive emails from prospective patients who have an X-ray or MRI they want to send us. Sometimes they want an opinion to back up a surgical recommendation; sometimes they want an opinion to support their desire to avoid surgery. In either case, when I tell them that the X-ray or MRI may not be telling the truth about their pain source, they become surprised and confused.

New findings say that many MRIs are useless. Investigators examined patients who had had an MRI for knee pain to determine whether the MRI was helpful in determining the final outcome of treatment.

Doctors examining the MRIs made the following recommendations for the 185 patients in the study:

- 39% of the MRIs were useful—mostly for sports injuries where a clear-cut defect could be seen.
- 18% were too equivocal for a determination to be made one way or another.
- 43% were judged "arguably useless." For the most part, patients in this group had nonspecific knee pain.[105]

Doctors report that the accuracy of ultrasound examination has been demonstrated by the high reliability of this method in the diagnosis of lateral meniscus lesions of the knee. They believe that ultrasound is a useful clinical tool for diagnosing knee pathology,[106] and that it has both high reliability and excellent diagnostic accuracy.[107]

In my own practice, I have found ultrasound to be a valuable tool.

"Magnetic resonance imaging (MRI) has the highest sensitivity of all methods for the diagnosis of intra-articular knee injuries. In spite of this, its benefit for the decision-making algorithm is questionable."[108]

In other words, an MRI may show a defect in the knee that may not actually be the source of the pain. The decision to have surgery based solely on this evidence could therefore be a mistake. In addition, because MRIs are overly sensitive, they may show "defects" that don't actually exist.

Researchers examined the medical records of patients who had undergone knee arthroscopy during 2008 and 2009, and who had had a preoperative MRI examination. The patients had lateral meniscus tears, anterior cruciate ligament (ACL) tears, and articular chondral lesions, with the diagnostic value of MRI the lowest for cartilage damage.

The researchers concluded: "There is no consensus regarding the role of MRI in the diagnosis of intra-articular lesions of the knee. To a certain extent, its use is related to local conditions. It can be concluded that MRI examination is not currently as important for the diagnosis of knee injuries as expected by both medical and lay communities."[109]

These opinions have been shared by others: "Although knee radiographs are widely considered as the gold standard for the assessment of knee osteoarthritis in clinical and scientific settings, they increasingly have significant limitations in situations when resolution and assessment of cartilage is required."[110]

In another study, not only was the cartilage diagnosis questioned, but the diagnoses of meniscal and ligament damage were as well, again in agreement with the research cited above. Researchers found that "[MRIs provided] a false positive rate of 65% for the medial meniscus, 43% for the lateral meniscus, 47.2% for the anterior cruciate ligament (treatment), and 41.7% for articular cartilage disease when compared with surgical findings."[111]

In other words, in these cases the patient was surgically opened, and the "defect" was not found to be present.

The conclusion is obvious: the "objective" evidence of technology-based tools—MRIs, X-rays, and other advanced diagnostic techniques—may contribute greatly to promoting cases of unnecessary or even ill-advised surgery. The end result? More pain for the recipients of these surgeries.

It is perfectly okay to question your MRI readings, especially since surgery may be unnecessary or even cause more damage.

"Bone-on-Bone" Arthritis

Many of my patients present with a diagnosis of "bone-on-bone arthritis," terminology used to describe a knee that has lost all cartilage to cushion the bones. Few actually have true "bone on bone." If the joint moves, there is typically cartilage present since cartilage is the slippery surface on the end of the bones that allow range of motion.

When the doctor says you have bone-on-bone arthritis, it may be used as an umbrella term to describe various levels of knee degeneration. In the knee joint, cartilage covers the tibia, femur, and the back of the kneecap (the patella); in addition to cartilage, there is the meniscus, which is the fibrous padding between the bones. A healthy knee glides efficiently and painlessly on these structures.

Bone-on-bone can mean that some or all of the cartilage and/or the meniscus have worn down or have defects, thereby causing the bones to rub together. Another diagnostic term that may refer to bone-on-bone is "osteochondral defect." The term "osteochondral" refers to the cartilage and bone as a unit. Patients often assume that bone-on-bone or an osteochondral defect means extreme and advanced cartilage deterioration, which is not usually the case.

Joint space, the space between the bones, is a challenge to surgeons. If there is no space between the bones, i.e, the cartilage has worn down—surgery cannot restore it. The philosophy then is to manage the knee pain as long as possible (often with repeated steroid injections that temporarily reduce pain, but eventually destroy whatever cartilage is left) prior to the knee replacement surgery.

Stem Cells Instead of Knee Replacement

In recent research, doctors followed patients for five years and found that five years after treatment, knees treated with stem cells were still better than before treatment.[112] In another study, doctors in China

Anatomy of the Knee Joint

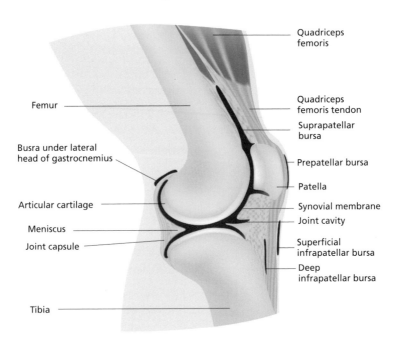

Quadriceps femoris

Femur

Quadriceps femoris tendon

Suprapatellar bursa

Busra under lateral head of gastrocnemius

Prepatellar bursa

Patella

Articular cartilage

Synovial membrane

Joint cavity

Meniscus

Superficial infrapatellar bursa

Joint capsule

Deep infrapatellar bursa

Tibia

announced that in their animal studies, stem cells injected into the site of a bone fracture promoted rapid and accelerated bone healing.[113]

Stem Cells for Bone Repair

Implications of the above research can help revolutionize the way standardized medicine addresses problems of bone degeneration and necrosis (bone death).

Researchers are looking at the osteoblasts, specialized mesenchyme-derived (stem) cells that account for bone synthesis, remodeling, and healing. What they are finding is that these cells rebuild bones through various mechanisms, including cell "homing" or "signaling," in which stem cells communicate with the surrounding tissue to help them navigate to the site of the wound and differentiate themselves into the material to build bone.[114] Other research suggests positive results even in cases of avascular necrosis.[115] Researchers in China announced that in their animal studies, stem cell injections accelerated bone healing, and that further research should investigate stem cell injections for fractures of the bone.[116]

PRP for Knee Osteoarthritis

Recently, numerous studies have appeared on the effectiveness of PRP in treating knee osteoarthritis.

In new research, doctors found that in a follow-up of one year or less, patients who had received PRP injections had improved functional outcomes when compared to those who had been given either hyaluronic acid or placebo.[117]

PRP seems to be more effective than hyaluronic acid in younger, active patients with low-grade osteoarthritis.[118]

In the medical journal *International Orthopaedics*, researchers showed that PRP enhances and accelerates the tendon healing process.[119]

Doctors say intra-articular multiple and single platelet-rich plasma (PRP) injections work as well as or better than hyaluronic acid (HA) injections in different stages of osteoarthritis of the knee.[120]

PRP helps regenerate degenerated bone in bone-on-bone knees.[121]

A Brief Outline of Other Treatments

The American Association of Family Physicians recently published a study titled *Nonsurgical Management of Knee Pain in Adults*. Following is an excerpt:

> The role of the family physician in managing knee pain is expanding as recent literature supports nonsurgical management for many patients. Here are nonsurgical recommendations:
>
> Oral analgesics—most commonly, nonsteroidal anti-inflammatory drugs and acetaminophen—are used initially in combination with physical therapy to manage the most typical causes of chronic knee pain.
>
> The American Academy of Orthopaedic Surgeons recommends against glucosamine/chondroitin supplementation for osteoarthritis as primary care.
>
> In patients who are not candidates for surgery, opioid analgesics should be used only if conservative pharmacotherapy is ineffective.
>
> Tears of the anterior cruciate ligament (ACL) are very frequent injuries, particularly in young and active people. Arthroscopic reconstruction using tendon auto- or allo-graft represents the gold standard for the management of ACL tears.
>
> Interestingly, the ACL has the potential to heal using intensive non-surgical rehabilitation procedures.
>
> Several biological factors influence this healing process as local intraligamentous cytokines (healing growth factors within the ligament) and mainly cell repair mechanisms controlled by stem cells or progenitor cells (a cell that can morph itself into something else that aids in repair).
>
> Understanding the mechanisms of this regeneration process and the cells involved may pave the way for novel, less invasive and biology-based strategies for ACL repair.[122]

Case Study of Patient with Ruptured ACL

Understanding how an ACL heals—even a complete rupture—has led doctors to turn their attention to biomaterials (blood platelets and stem cells). One of the things doctors are looking at is "scaffolding," a surgical procedure in which a cartilage patch is placed over a cartilage defect and then "pasted in" with PRP or stem cell gel. However, in some instances the body may make its own scaffolding out of pooled blood and use this blood as the foundation to regenerate a ligament—even a completely ruptured ACL.

Doctors shared a case history of a 12-year-old boy who was hit by a car and suffered a grievous knee injury. The boy was also a high-level hockey player. What makes this story so amazing is that the knee damage was so severe in terms of broken bones, that surgery to reconstruct the ACL had to be postponed until the bones could heal first (he had two surgeries right after the accident related to the bone damage). *When doctors operated 16 months later to reconstruct the ACL, they found it to be completely regenerated.*

The doctors were baffled, since this should not have happened. The medical literature states that a completely ruptured ACL does not heal, because blood and healing cells cannot reach it.

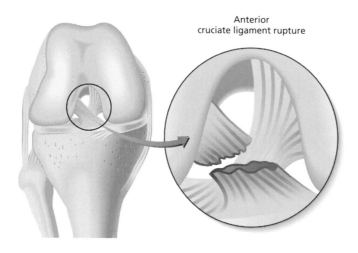

Anterior
cruciate ligament rupture

Yet, their patient with traumatic knee injury with multiple ruptured ligaments healed over the course of 16 months.

It is likely that bracing associated with the patient's second surgery and delayed union of his tibial fracture allowed healing tissue to be protected from excessive stress until it remodeled with sufficient strength. It is possible that intra-articular scar formation contributed to his healing capacity—possibly the blood scaffold.

Twenty months after the accident, the boy returned to playing competitive hockey—and two and a half years later, he was still playing, with no adverse effects to his knee.[123]

In the above scenario and in the surgical procedure, the common factor in ACL healing is time. However, many active people do not have the time to rehab. This lack of patience creates more surgery. In anterior cruciate ligament reconstruction, the overall incidence rate of having to repeat the surgery within 24 months is six times greater than for someone who has never had an ACL tear.

The case study above was presented at the 2013 annual meeting of the American Orthopaedic Society for Sports Medicine (AOSSM).

Doctors have found that within 24 months of anterior cruciate ligament reconstruction, female athletes had a rate of injury more than four times greater than their healthy counterparts.

Researchers looked at 78 patients (59 female, 19 male) between 10 and 25 years of age who underwent anterior cruciate ligament reconstruction, with 47 healthy controls. Each ACL reconstruction subject was followed for injury and athletic exposure for a 24-month period after returning to play.

Twenty-three of the ACL reconstruction individuals and four control subjects suffered an ACL injury during the 24-month period. In the ACL group, there also appeared to be a trend for female subjects to be two times more likely to suffer an injury on the *opposite* knee than on the previously injured one.

Overall, 29.5% of athletes suffered a second ACL injury within 24 months of returning to activity, with 20.5% sustaining an opposite leg injury and 9.0% incurring a graft re-tear injury on the same leg. A higher proportion of females (23.7%) suffered an opposite leg injury compared to males (10.5%).

In a 2015 study, doctors addressed the epidemic of anterior cruciate ligament injuries among young athletes, as well as the large number of patients who have had ACL reconstruction surgery and then undergo a second knee operation.

"This is the first study to evaluate, on a population level, the percentage of patients under age 21 who had subsequent ACL or non-ACL knee surgery following a primary anterior cruciate ligament reconstruction," said pediatric orthopedic surgeon Emily Dodwell, lead investigator of the study by researchers at the Hospital for Special Surgery in New York City.

"The increasing rate of ACL injuries is concerning, although not surprising, given greater participation in sports," Dr. Dodwell said. The study noted that children are starting sports at a younger age, playing for longer durations with greater intensity, and often concentrating on a single sport year-round, resulting in overuse and acute injuries. "For young people who have primary surgery to reconstruct a torn ACL, it is troubling that they have relatively high rates of subsequent ACL reconstruction or surgery for another knee injury. Further research is needed to determine factors associated with subsequent injury and surgery so we can implement strategies to keep our youth safe while engaging in sports." [124]

ACL RUPTURE PREVENTION

The internet is filled with articles on how to prevent ACL tears. Various suggestions include strength training, aerobic training, nutrition, coordination exercises, balance and posture, knee bracing, etc. But what about the high-risk knee, one that has already been compromised by wear and tear and previous injury? Is there a way to prevent ACL injury when you're already at high risk? How about avoiding the first surgery!!!

THE LIGAMENT

If you look at a full-color picture of human anatomy, you will see that muscles are big and that they are red, which results from the abundant

Knee Sprain
(right knee, front view)

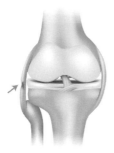 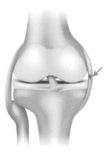 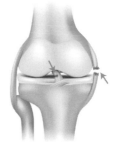

Torn lateral collateral ligament (LCL)	Torn medial collateral ligament (MCL)	Torn medial collateral ligament (MCL) and anterior cruciate ligament (ACL)

blood supply that runs through them to help them grow and repair. Ligaments, on the other hand, are small and white and resemble thick rubber bands. They do not have an abundant blood supply, and as a result they usually do not heal well from injury. Prior to regenerative medicine, ligament tears often required surgery.

Over the course of an athlete's season, ligaments may become weaker and lose elasticity, becoming more prone to injury. At this point, pain, soreness, and loss of strength may occur in the knee.

Icing, anti-inflammatory medications, and knee bracing or taping are treatments used to get the player through the season. *However, it is possible that these remedies actually increase the risk of ACL tear rather than preventing it.* This observation is supported by many medical papers citing the pros and cons of knee bracing and taping and the circulatory and healing disruptions caused by icing.

Further, the player begins to overcompensate for the painful knee, and in doing so puts the "healthy knee" at greater risk for severe ACL damage. In addition, chronic ankle sprains have been cited as a cause of higher risk to ACL tear.

THE TREATMENT CAUSES INJURY

One thing that the treatments described above have in common is that they weaken ligaments. Icing, as stated, disrupts the circulation needed to bring the healing cells to damaged ligaments. Anti-inflammatory medications increase the risk of ligament damage by suppressing immune function and blocking the synthesis of collagen. There is no conclusive evidence that knee braces block injury, and in fact, their use may "trick" the athlete into a comfort level of believeing their knee to be protected when, in fact, it is not. The treatment causes the injury.

To PREVENT DEVASTATING ACL injuries, athletes need to look into treatment with biomedicine to regrow and strengthen their ligaments—as we have seen throughout this book, those treatments are Stem Cell Therapy, Platelet-Rich Plasma (PRP) Therapy, and Prolotherapy.

In 2009, Prolotherapy doctors published a case history of a patient with a complete ACL rupture. The patient was an 18-year-old female who sustained a right knee injury during a downhill skiing accident. MRI revealed a high-grade partial rupture versus a complete rupture. The patient deferred surgical treatment. At 21 weeks post-injury, with unstable gait and an inability to climb stairs, she consented to undergo Prolotherapy injections. She received seven Prolotherapy sessions over a 15-week period. At-home exercises were initiated at the third session. The results were that the patient improved: walking on flat ground improved 4 weeks after initiation of Prolotherapy, and she could ride a stationary bicycle for half an hour by 12 weeks. By 15 weeks, the patient had no instability climbing and descending stairs, the anterior drawer test was negative, and MRI showed an intact ACL with fibrosis. Subsequently, she returned to full sport activity.[125]

This was not the only documented research on ACL repair and Prolotherapy. Doctors found that in patients with symptomatic anterior cruciate ligament laxity and weakening, intermittent Prolotherapy injections resulted in clinically and statistically significant improvement in ACL laxity, pain, swelling, and knee range of motion.[126]

5

Back Pain

MRI Is Sending People to Surgery Who Don't Need It

All too frequently, a medical study comes across my desk that says patients are too often choosing to have elective orthopedic surgery. In a recent paper, doctors found that *more than 50% of the patients would have a spinal surgery if their doctor told them they had an abnormal spinal MRI, even if they had no pain or restricted movement.*

The authors surmised that patients overemphasize the value of MRIs and have mixed perceptions of the relative risk and effectiveness of surgical intervention compared with more conservative management.[127]

Doctors analyzed the most frequently cited papers in lumbar spine surgery and measured their impact on the entire lumbar spine literature. Here is what they found: The most cited paper was "the classic paper" from 1990 that described magnetic resonance imaging (MRI) findings in individuals without back pain, sciatica, and neurogenic claudication (impairment), showing that spinal stenosis and herniated discs can be incidentally found when scanning patients.[128] The word "incidental" meant that the patient had no pain. The purpose of the paper was to examine why people with no back pain show abnormalities on MRI.

More than a quarter of a century later, doctors are still citing the paper and asking the same question: "Why does this patient have clear problems on MRI but no back pain?" And the secondary question: "Should we send this patient to surgery?"

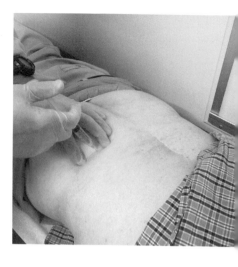

The second most cited (and far more recent) study similarly showed that patients who had no symptoms of back pain who underwent lumbar spine magnetic resonance imaging frequently had lumbar degeneration and disease.[129]

The two most cited research papers in relationship to spinal surgery are studies on why patients had absolute and clear spinal problems on MRI and yet showed no signs of pain or expressed any problems.[130]

I often see patients who have severe back pain and show me an MRI, X-ray, and/or scan that was inconclusive. For instance, a patient can have muscle spasm from a simple back strain, which can cause excruciating pain and may limit the ability to walk or even stand. Conversely, a large herniated disc may be completely painless. Yet the patient with the large herniated disc may be sent to surgery. *Why do we see so many failed back surgery patients?* Because lower back pain is one of the most difficult complaints to accurately diagnose and treat. The reason for the insurance diagnosis code of "Failed Back Surgery Syndrome" is that so many back surgeries fail.

As the research above has shown, magnetic resonance imaging (MRI) for back pain remains controversial because a considerable proportion of patients may be classified incorrectly by MRI for lumbar disc herniation and spinal stenosis.

Not only that, but doctors writing in the *European Journal of Pain* reported that while the importance of MRI findings remains controversial, best evidence does not support the use of any prognostic test in clinical practice in selecting patients for lumbar spinal fusion.

This supports recent findings that despite doctors frequently requesting MRIs for the lumbar spine, the imaging performs poorly and is not likely to identify the anatomical structures that are the source of pain.[131] This is why a physical examination, *not* an MRI, is the main diagnostic tool I employ. While MRI is used as an ancillary confirmation, it is most often wrong when used solely on its own as a diagnostic tool.[132]

Recently, doctors in Canada found that more than half of lower-back MRIs ordered at two Canadian hospitals were either inappropriate or of questionable value for patients.

And family doctors were more likely to order these unnecessary tests compared to other specialists. The findings are important, because in some parts of Canada, MRI tests for the lower back account for about one-third of all MRI requests. Across the country, wait times for MRIs are long, and patient access is limited.[133]

From another study from the University of Connecticut Health Center: "More than 85% of patients seen at primary care practices have low back pain that cannot be attributed to a specific disease or an anatomic abnormality, and it is well known that imaging of

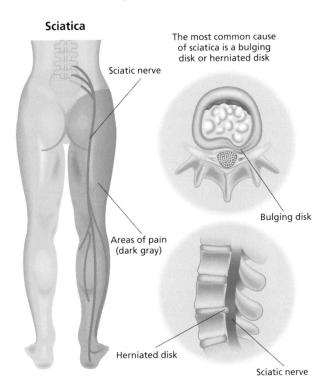

Sciatica

Sciatic nerve

The most common cause of sciatica is a bulging disk or herniated disk

Bulging disk

Areas of pain (dark gray)

Herniated disk

Sciatic nerve

asymptomatic patients often reveals anatomic abnormalities, such as herniated discs. One of the risks of routinely imaging uncomplicated acute low back pain is patient 'labeling'; no evidence exists that labeling patients with low back pain with a specific anatomic diagnosis improves outcomes."[134]

This evidence confirms that clinicians should refrain from routine, immediate lumbar imaging in patients with nonspecific, acute or subacute lower back pain with no indications of underlying serious conditions. Specific consideration of patient expectations about the value of imaging was not addressed here; however, this aspect must be considered to avoid unnecessary MRI imaging while also meeting patient expectations and increasing patient satisfaction."[135]

In another recent paper, researchers concluded that at present, *best evidence does not support the use of any prognostic test in clinical practice in selecting patients for lumbar spinal fusion.*[136]

But MRI *Is* Suggesting Fusion Surgery for Sacroiliac Joint Dysfunction—Shouldn't I Get the Surgery?

In one research paper, doctors concluded that sacroiliac joint spinal fusion for the management of chronic lower back pain is "murky," and that the consequences of the unsupported enthusiasm for surgical management of disc-related back pain negatively impacts the public perception of spinal surgeons.[137]

There is a further double jeopardy for patients—new research questions whether or not MRI has any value in determining sciatica treatment or diagnosis.[138] We now have a possibly misleading MRI sending a patient for a procedure that may not work, causing the patient more problems.

As noted in the above recent study, researchers have shown that diagnosis of sacroiliac joint dysfunction is flawed.[139, 140] This misdiagnosis is why doctors say that the sacroiliac joint spinal fusion for the management of chronic lower back pain is "murky" and can lead to Failed Back Surgery Syndrome.

One of my patients is a woman in her early seventies. She presented with her husband after not one, but two sacral fusions, one on the right and one on the left. You might be appalled if you saw the amount of metal that was used to do the fusion. Huge screws, too. Because of continued pain on the left side, her surgeon wanted her to redo the left fusion. She came to me for advice.

During examination, I pressed on her gluteus muscles, away from the fusion site and she winced in pain. I immediately told her that her pain was not coming from the sacroiliac joint, and that she simply had a strain where the muscles were attached to the pelvis. I asked her if the surgeon actually examined this area and to my astonishment, her answer was, "no." She and her husband looked like deer in headlights, confused as to what I was telling them. How could her pain not be related to the joint, and the subsequent fusion, when she had surgery for that issue. I told them I was sorry, but the surgery never needed to be done if this is where the pain had been. It took about a half hour for them to digest this information, and we proceeded to inject PRP though the muscles down to the bone interface. We call that the enthesis. She returned two weeks later, and was about 50% better. I injected again, and expect full recovery with one more series of injections.

This is the most common scenario in my office. Not necessarily the same area, but almost all areas of the body. Please remember, elective surgery means you, the patient, get to elect whether or not to proceed to surgery. It is your body. You own it. You decide, not the doctor.

If It Isn't the Discs, Then What *Is* Causing Your Back Pain?

A recent study in the medical journal *Pain Medicine* questions the prevailing thought that discs are a major culprit in back issues. The researchers wrote: "Between 26% and 42% of chronic low back pain is attributed to internal disc disruption of lumbar intervertebral discs (i.e., a disc problem in the lower back). These prevalence estimates and data characterizing discogenic pain originate largely from research

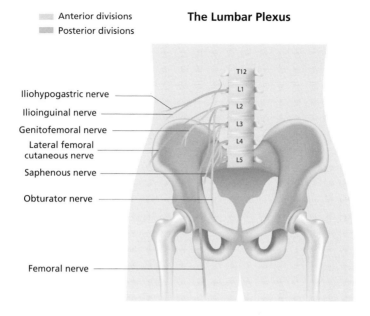

The Lumbar Plexus

Anterior divisions
Posterior divisions

Iliohypogastric nerve

Ilioinguinal nerve

Genitofemoral nerve

Lateral femoral
cutaneous nerve

Saphenous nerve

Obturator nerve

Femoral nerve

T12
L1
L2
L3
L4
L5

conducted 20 years ago. With few studies since, their concordance with rates in community practice has rarely been addressed."

The researchers had some doubts about these numbers. In conducting their own tests, they found that discogenic pain was not as prevalent but was still within the confidence intervals previously reported (meaning in the ballpark), owing to the fact that they discovered discs as being responsible for pain 21% of the time.[141]

If this is the case, then it can be said that something else is causing your back pain 79% of the time.

As we have discussed, one of the great challenges in treating back pain is identifying the source of the patient's pain. As I indicated above, the majority of patients believe that the source of their pain has been identified by their MRI. However, in many patients the picture of disc degeneration is not an accurate profile of the cause of pain. Most often, I find that it is the spinal ligaments that are involved—in other words, the pain is being caused by a simple "sprain." I ask patients whether they have ever had a sprained ankle. Most say yes, and that it hurt quite a bit. I then tell them that they have the equivalent of a sprained "ankle" in their back, and nothing more, regardless of what the MRI or other films show. Do people get surgery for a sprained ankle? Of course not!! This is not to say that surgery may be needed for a tendon or ligament rupture, or fracture.

This is difficult for people to understand, because they see their MRI with an apparently "obvious" abnormality that requires surgical intervention. However, once they have had a physical examination and are shown where the pain is being generated, patients come to understand that their back pain may be based on ligament irritation at the point where the ligaments attach to bone (enthesopathy). A treatment plan with realistic expectations can then be discussed using Stem Cell Therapy or Platelet-Rich Plasma Therapy.

All too often, patients with failed back surgery syndrome tell me that their surgeon never gave them a physical examination, but simply recommended surgery based on a diagnostic film.

Doctors at the Mayo Clinic now agree that before treatments are initiated for back pain, a thorough examination of the spinal ligaments is needed.

These doctors were able to recommend guidelines in monitoring patient movement (especially side-to- side bending) as indications of when discs were the problem and when spinal ligaments were, allowing for more precise treatment strategies.[142] Determination of the diagnosis is dependent on a physical examination, not an MRI.

Spinal Disc Herniation

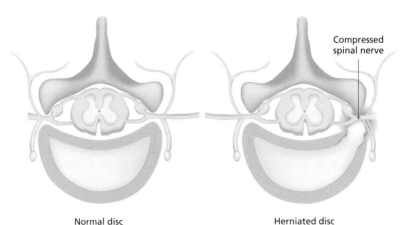

Compressed
spinal nerve

Normal disc   Herniated disc

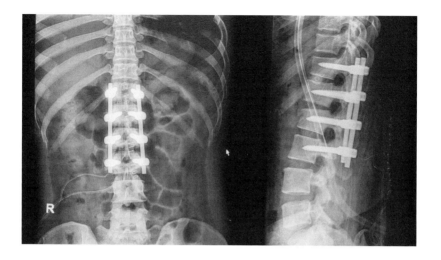

"Failed back surgery syndrome is a complication of spine surgery that leads to chronic pain and disability, often with disastrous emotional consequences to the patient." (Romero-Vargas S, Obil-Chavarria C, Zárate-Kalfopolus B, Rosales-Olivares LM, Alpizar-Aguirre A, Reyes-Sánchez AA. Profile of the patient with failed back surgery syndrome in the National Institute of Rehabilitation. Comparative analysis. Cir Cir. 2015 Mar-Apr;83(2):117-23. doi: 10.1016/j.circir.2015.04.006. Epub 2015 May 16.)

In a study of 65 patients, 18 (group I) had their first spine surgeries performed at the researchers' institution, and the other 47 patients (group II) had their first surgeries performed at another hospital.

Among those in Group I, the majority had had a previous diagnosis of lumbar stenosis, whereas disc herniation was the main diagnosis in group II. The main cause of failed back surgery syndrome in Group I was technical error during surgery (61.1%), while in Group II this cause represented only 6.3% of the syndrome. Among the patients in this latter group, misdiagnosis was highly prevalent (57.4%).[143]

A Note on Epidural Steroid Injections

Epidural steroid injection is the most frequently performed pain procedure. It is becoming clear that epidural steroid injections for various spinal conditions are best used for a patient who is in pain and waiting for back surgery. If you have decided that you are getting a spinal surgery, then an epidural may be the procedure you want prior to surgery.

Doctors find that epidural steroid injections provide modest pain relief for up to 3 months in patients with lumbosacral radicular pain caused by herniated discs, but they have no impact on physical disability or incidence of surgery.[144]

In another study, the immediate response to transforaminal epidural steroid injection was approximately 80%. However, transforaminal epidural steroid injection cannot alter the need for surgery in the long term.[145]

A third study concluded that while nearly 20% of patients had spinal surgery after one steroid injection, the ones who did were at least able to reduce the number of pain medications they had been on prior to the surgery.[146] The study did not measure those needing painkillers after the surgery.

As pointed out by Thomas Jefferson University, Rothman Institute researchers, for some, the epidural steroid injections did not work at all. "Patients with lumbar disc herniation treated with epidural steroid injection had no improvement in short- or long-term outcomes compared with patients who were not treated with epidural steroid injection."[147]

In a review published in the medical journal *Spine*, epidural steroid injections were not only questioned for lack of effectiveness, but also called dangerous: "[Epidural steroid injections] are typically short-acting and ineffective over the longer term, while exposing patients to major risks/complications . . . . Although the benefits for epidural steroid injections may include transient pain relief for those with/without surgical disease, the multitude of risks attributed to these injections outweighs the benefits." [148]

Epidural Steroid Injection Side Effects

Epidural steroid injections are given to reduce inflammation in the nerves that pass through the spinal canal. Many pain management specialists believe that nerve inflammation is the root cause of the patient's discomfort and the cause of radiating pain and numbness down the patient's legs. Patients with these problems are often diagnosed as having "sciatica," a term used to describe injury or compression of the sciatic nerve.

Research published in the medical journal *Physical medicine and rehabilitation clinics of North America* suggests: "Epidural steroid injection has been used as a treatment for low back pain for over 50 years. In the last 10 to 15 years, there has been a significant increase in [their use] for the treatment of low back pain and radicular pain without clear improvements in outcomes." [149]

As an orthopedic pain specialist, I see many patients with radiating lower back pain. When I first examine these patients, I find that many of them have been diagnosed with sciatica. On examination, however, I find that many of these patients do not have sciatica at all—and so of course epidural steroid injections have failed them. Typically, the pain these patients are suffering is not from nerve impingement. To me, when an epidural fails, that is good news for the patient.

Patients Afraid to Move Nearly Three Years After Surgery

Patients with back pain have many common concerns. One is that they are afraid to move because of the pain. Surgery is supposed to take care of this fear. Researchers followed 97 patients after their disc surgery, looking for a postsurgical occurrence of kinesiophobia (fear of movement). What they found was surprising.

The researchers reported:

"Half of the patients suffered from kinesiophobia 10-34 months after surgery for disc herniation.

These patients were more disabled, had more pain, more catastrophizing thoughts, more symptoms of depression, lower self-efficacy, and poorer health-related quality of life than patients without kinesiophobia." [150]

For many, surgery did not quell their fears but in fact made them worse.

Because of these fears, doctors began examining a cognitive behavioral-based physical therapy, where a physical therapist would intervene and change the therapy strategies to address fears.

Unfortunately, one study suggested that another problem be addressed—"[t]hat physical therapists self-perceive a lack of knowledge, skills, and time to provide this intervention."[151]

Research suggests that a targeted cognitive behavioral-based physical therapy program may result in significant and clinically meaningful improvement in postoperative outcomes. It has the potential to be an evidence-based program that clinicians can recommend for patients who are at risk for poor recovery following spine surgery.[152]

Why Do Doctors Send Patients at Risk for Poor Recovery to Spine Surgery?

When I was in medical school, I did surgical research and assisted in the operating room much more than my classmates. By the time I had finished medical school and internship (where I spent as much time as possible doing orthopedic procedures), I had seen too many surgical failures, including my own shoulder surgery. And worse, when the first surgery clearly failed, the patient was offered a *second* surgery to fix the first one. Older patients usually refused the second surgery, later documented in the research: "The likelihood of repeat surgery for spinal stenosis declined with increasing age and other diseases, perhaps because of concern for greater risks."[153] There may have been fewer surgeries because older patients were not able to have them— probably a blessing in disguise.

Informing Patients of Back Surgery Risk

From the medical journal *Spine*: "Patients should be informed that the likelihood of reoperation following a lumbar spine operation is substantial."[154]

From the medical journal: Orthopedic Reviews: "Multilevel fusion for degenerative disease still has a high rate of complications, up

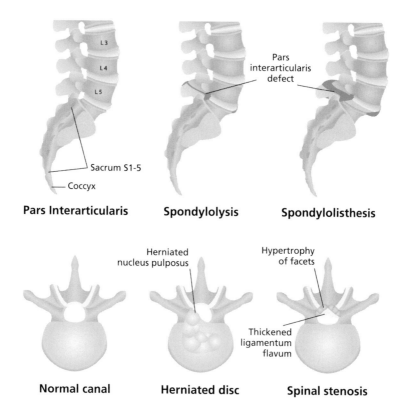

Pars Interticularis

L3
L4
L5

Sacrum S1-5
Coccyx

Spondylolysis

Pars interarticularis defect

Spondylolisthesis

Normal canal

Herniated nucleus pulposus

Herniated disc

Hypertrophy of facets

Thickened ligamentum flavum

Spinal stenosis

to 50%. The problem of adjacent segment disease after fusion surgery has not yet been solved." [155] The segment above the fusion and the one below then take the brunt of the movement stresses and often break down.

Biomaterials for Treating Spinal Instability Instead of Surgery

Persistent or chronic lower back pain usually develops over an extended period of time due to interacting causative factors involving the vertebrae and their supporting tissues.

Although these two types of "extended pain" are similar in many respects, researchers have distinguished them according to a few basic guidelines.

Generally, pain is described as "persistent" if it does not heal promptly, based on statistical standards, or if it recurs regularly, in defiance of any treatments provided. "Chronic" is the term usually reserved for pain lasting longer than three months; in both cause and effect, chronic pain often involves psychological as well as physical factors. Acute pain is defined as that lasting less than three months.

Recently, more doctors have been discussing regenerative medicine for problems of the spine, especially when damaged spinal ligaments are causing spinal instability or enthesopathy (areas of irritable ligament attachment to bone). Among these treatments are Stem Cell Therapy and Platelet-Rich Plasma Therapy (PRP), which doctors say may lead to an entirely new method of treating back pain patients.

Spinal Ligaments

The chronic lower back pain patient typically experiences some type of trauma or overuse to the lower back that causes injury to the iliolumbar, interspinous, and supraspinous ligaments, the ligaments that hold the pelvis to the vertebrae and spinal processes in place. Ligaments are designed to handle a normal amount of stress that stretches them to their natural limit, returning to their normal length once the stress is removed. If additional (traumatic) stress is applied, stretching the ligament beyond its natural range of extension, the ligament does not return to its normal length but instead remains permanently overstretched, diminishing its integrity and attachment to the bone.

Unlike muscle tissue, ligaments and tendons have a very limited circulatory system and a poor supply of blood to regenerate them. This is why ligaments may not heal and instead can remain in a weakened and irritable inflammatory state.

Here is a remarkable statement from the medical journal *Spine*:

"As important as the vertebral ligaments are in maintaining the integrity of the spinal column and protecting the contents of the spinal canal, a single detailed review of their anatomy and function is missing in the literature." [156]

PRP for Back Pain

Research has shown Platelet-Rich Plasma Therapy (PRP) to be effective in treating degenerative disc disease by addressing the problems of spinal ligament instability and stimulating the regeneration of the discs indirectly (discs were not injected directly but showed an increase in disc height).[157] The same research cites that as in any medicine, the sooner the degeneration is addressed, the better the results in patient satisfaction. PRP is no exception. "The administration of PRP has a protective effect on damaged discs in the acute and delayed injection settings representing clinical treatment with PRP in the early versus late stages of the degenerative process. It appears that earlier intervention in the disease process would be more beneficial than PRP treatment of already severely degenerated discs."[157]

Research presented by international scientists in Italy in 2015 showed that PRP is able to recover the mechanical properties of denatured discs, thereby providing a promising effective therapeutic modality.[158]

In fact, doctors now think that stress on the ligaments may be the cause for most pain in degenerative disc disease, confirming earlier research from 2010. [159]

PRP is an effective means of alleviating back pain because it eliminates pain by healing the underlying issue. As the research above points out, PRP can eliminate the need for surgery.

6

Hip Pain

Recently a new paper suggested that the treatment of hip osteoarthritis, like those of other joint osteoarthritic problems, is redefining itself at a pace probably not seen since the advent of hip replacement surgery. Some doctors are upset that patients are not given the full story on hip replacement options and alternatives. Despite the availability of evidence-based guidelines for conservative treatment of osteoarthritis, management of degenerated joints is often confined to the use of painkillers and the wait for eventual total joint replacement. This suggests a gap in knowledge for those with osteoarthritis regarding the many different treatment options available to them.[160]

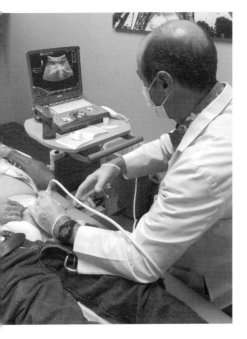

How wide a gap? One study says that when given time and educational materials to deliberate whether or not to proceed with hip replacement, more patients decide not to have surgery.[161]

Research such as this makes clear that people with hip osteoarthritis are too often told only about hip replacement as a treatment, so they do not even know about the nonsurgical treatments available.

Here is what researchers said: "Conservative treatment modalities in osteoarthritis of hip or knee are underused, whereas the demand for surgery is rising substantially. To improve the use of conservative treatments, a more in-depth understanding of the reasons for patients' treatment choice is required. This study identifies the reasons for choice of treatment in patients with hip or knee osteoarthritis.

Various treatment options were discussed: medication, exercise, physical therapy, injections, surgery, complementary and alternative treatment. Four key themes underlying the choice for or against a treatment were identified:

1. treatment characteristics: expectations about its effectiveness and risks, the degree to which it can be personalized to a patient's needs and wishes, and the accessibility of a treatment;
2. personal investment: in terms of money and time;
3. personal circumstances: age, body weight, comorbidities and previous experience with a treatment; and
4. support and advice: from the patient's social environment and healthcare providers."[162]

The feeling is that hip replacement or arthroscopic surgery is readily available. There is an expectation that surgery fixes everything and improves general overall health. There is a lot of expectation. Yet other research says these expectations are not met, and this is clearly cause for concern.

Presenting alternatives to hip replacement surgery is an important function in the patient–doctor relationship, as suggested in this recent study:

"Arthroscopic surgery is commonly performed in the knee, shoulder, elbow, and hip. However, the role it plays in the management of osteoarthritis is controversial. Routine arthroscopic management of osteoarthritis was once common, but this

Total Hip Replacement

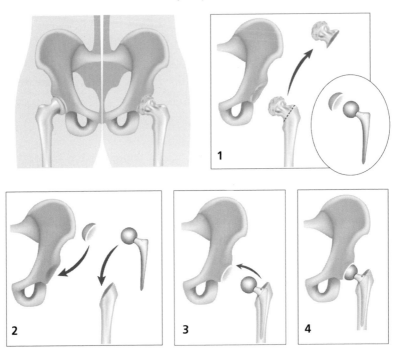

practice has been recently scrutinized. Although some believe that there is no role for arthroscopic treatment in the management of osteoarthritis, it may be appropriate and beneficial in certain situations. The clinical success of such treatment may be rooted in appropriate patient selection and adherence to a specific surgical technique. Arthroscopy may serve as an effective and less invasive option than traditional methods of managing osteoarthritis."[163]

In other words, as controversial and unproven as arthroscopic surgery is, it may still be better than hip replacement.

Far better than both as a first option, in my opinion, are the biomedicine treatments of Stem Cell Therapy and Platelet-Rich Plasma (PRP) Therapy.

Treating Hip Osteoarthritis

Can Stem Cell Therapy and Platelet-Rich Plasma Therapy be effective in treating hip osteoarthritis and in helping you avoid a hip replacement surgery? The answer in many cases is yes. However, success is dependent on a physical examination and a practice of best diagnosis. The hip is a tricky and complex area filled with many pain generator suspects.

Diagnosing Hip Pain

In February 2012, research was presented at the American Orthopaedic Society for Sports Medicine's (AOSSM) Specialty Day meeting suggesting that when doctors treat people with hip pain, "Physicians should not replace clinical observation with the use of magnetic resonance images (MRI)." The research stated that when MRIs were

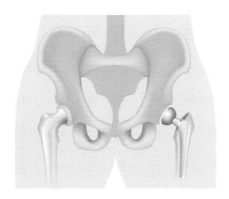

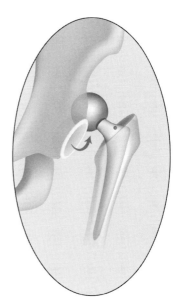

Dislocation after Total Hip Replacement Surgery

performed on volunteers *without* hip pain, *73% showed abnormal findings.*

Abnormal findings = surgical procedure.

This simple equation is well documented in the medical literature. Medical journals are filled with studies suggesting that while MRI is frequently used to diagnose conditions affecting the hip, its effectiveness in determining hip pain is not as valuable as a physical examination. And MRIs are not cost effective.[164]

In the medical journal *Pain Physician,* doctors agreed, and they offered a commentary that warned physicians that the true causes of hip pain can be easily overlooked and misdiagnosed because of the MRI.[165]

Misdiagnosed hip pain can lead to back surgery!

Not only might you get a hip replacement you may not need, you may in addition suffer a back surgery you don't need. Doctors have noted that the symptoms of hip pain and spinal stenosis leg pain can be very similar, with only subtle differences in both history and clinical examinations. Spinal stenosis is classically diagnosed in patients with leg pain that occurs during standing or walking and is relieved when the individual sits down. This is a clinical diagnosis that doctors say can only be confirmed by MRI.

However, in one paper, researchers showed that in *as many as 50% of elderly patients*, MRI gave a false positive diagnosis of spinal stenosis. Those MRI results might prompt a surgeon to perform spinal surgery. When the hip symptoms persist and remain undetected, it is even possible that a second unnecessary back surgery could be performed.

The following paper reported on patients who had MRI scans and multiple epidural injections and were subjected to repeat back surgeries, all while continuing to complain of their leg pain—the source of which was hip pathology.[166]

This is why some patients continue to experience hip pain after elective hip replacement surgery. One research study advised doctors to look for pain originating from different sources not directly linked to the replacement hardware, as something else must have been the problem.[167] This revelation comes a little late.

I see patients who were misdiagnosed and their pain generators overlooked. They have hip pain and an MRI in their chart showing a herniated disc in the lower back. After they had back surgery, the hip pain remained.

This chapter should provide a cautionary note for patients who insist that the MRI is providing the evidence needed to end their pain.

In one study of patients who received a hip replacement, researchers noted postoperative complications occurring in almost 20% of the patients. Dislocation was the most common complication, followed by wound infection.[168]

Included in those worries are fresh concerns about the amount of bone loss in the first surgery and the ability to perform a successful revision or future replacement surgery to replace worn-out hardware.[169]

Bone Defects and Bone Death

For some patients, bone defects in the hip represent a great challenge. When the protective cartilage wears away on the "ball" of the hip

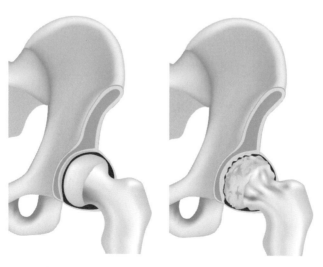

Healthy hip joint   **Osteoarthritis**

joint (the femoral head), there can be direct contact with the pelvic acetabulum (part of the pelvis bone in which the femur is seated). For some patients with advanced osteoarthritis or avascular necrosis (bone death) there may be the crunching and grinding of bone on bone.

FIXING THE FEMORAL HEAD MEANS REPLACEMENT

The most-used procedure does not fix the femoral head, instead replacing it (hip replacement) through amputation of the head of the femur and addition of prosthesis (total hip arthroplasty). Since not everyone is suitable for or wants to have the procedure, researchers are exploring ways to fix the femoral head before it becomes unstable or collapses and requires artificial joint replacement.

One method is to patch the bone defects—this is autologous bone grafting. Some of the bone is cut into a patch in the hope that it will take root and grow. However, the amount of bone available for grafting is quite limited as case histories point out.[170]

Regenerating the bone is an appealing remedy, leading researchers to look at Stem Cell Therapy, using one's own stem cells to heal bone defects. In recent research doctors suggested stem cells. The injection of stem cells into the joint can initiate the healing environment in the affected hip, including the regrowth of bone in cases of osteonecrosis (bone death).[171]

THE USE OF stem cells for the treatment of avascular necrosis (bone death due to interruption of the blood supply) of the femoral head presents a new and exciting remedial procedure.

In pre-clinical studies, the use of stem cells uniformly demonstrates improvements in osteogenesis (bone growth) and angiogenesis (blood vessel formation). In clinical studies, groups treated with stem cells have shown significant improvements in patient-reported outcomes.[172]

The Importance of Bone in Hip Replacement

The healing of hip osteoarthritis can be complex and complicated, especially if complex and complicated treatments are employed. Once

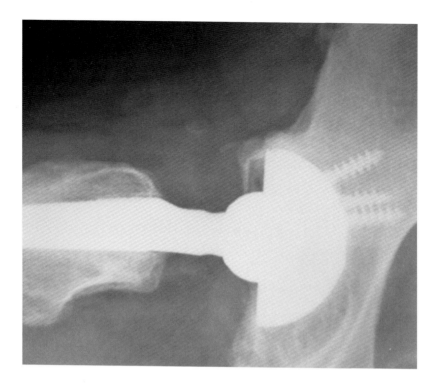

failed surgery exacerbates the matter, it is even more difficult to remedy the hip, especially as the patient ages.

The incidence of osteoarthritis is constantly advancing with increased longevity. Aging also leads to an increasing number of patients with osteoporosis (decreased bone mass) who "need" hip replacement for osteoarthritis. Osteoporosis has three major potential complications in total hip arthroplasty: perioperative (that is, near the time of the surgery) fracture, an increased risk of periprosthetic fracture (fracture of bones near the implant), and late aseptic loosening (loosening of hip replacement components). A study examining the effects of osteoporosis on total hip replacement procedure outcome highlights the importance of an adequate study of calcium-phosphorus metabolism in patients who are candidates for hip surgery, as well as the need to start a suitable therapy to recover the bone mass before surgery. Poor bone quality of the hip joint is an important risk factor limiting the durability and longevity of the hip replacement.[173]

However, if we are prepping the patient for hip replacement by strengthening the bone to hold the artificial devices, why not regrow the bone and cartilage and repair the tissue with the goal of avoiding surgery?

Research on Stem Cells and Platelet-Rich Plasma for Hip Repair

Platelet-rich plasma (PRP), obtained by withdrawing the patient's blood and concentrating the platelets, represents a safe, economical, easy to prepare, and easy to inject source of growth factors.

Platelets contain numerous growth factors, and a large number of them have specific activity in cartilage regeneration. PRP is able to significantly reduce pain and improve joint function.[174]

A study done in 2012 examined patient safety and symptomatic changes among 40 patients receiving Platelet-Rich Plasma (PRP) Therapy for osteoarthritis of the hip. In the study, each joint received three injections of PRP, administered once a week. The primary end point was meaningful pain relief, which was described as a reduction in pain intensity of at least 30% at six months post-treatment.

Secondary end points included reduction in the level of disability of at least 30% and the percentage of positive responders—that is, the number of patients who achieved a greater than 30% reduction in pain and disability.

The results were statistically significant reductions in pain and improvement in function as reported at seven weeks and again at six months.

Twenty-three patients (58%) reported a clinically relevant reduction of pain (45%). Sixteen (40%) of these patients were classified as excellent responders and showed an early pain reduction at six or seven weeks that was sustained at 6 months, accompanied by a parallel reduction of disability.[175]

From a January 2016 paper: "Results indicated that intra-articular PRP injections offer a significant clinical improvement in patients with hip osteoarthritis without relevant side effects."[176]

In other research, doctors followed patients who received Stem Cell Therapy for hip, knee, or ankle osteoarthritis and documented such therapeutic benefits as increased walking distance, increased function, and reduced pain.[177]

Patient Expectations Following Hip Resurfacing

Many times a patient will come into our office with a stack of MRIs, a post-surgical report, and a promise that they were told that they could resume their running after a hip resurfacing procedure. Unfortunately for them, the surgery did not meet their expectations. Recently published research in the American Journal of Sports Medicine, says "Running is possible after hip resurfacing, and runners can even return to some level of competition, but this short follow-up series of hip resurfacing in athletes should be interpreted with caution regarding implant survival."[178]

Lessen Your Expectations as to What Sports You Can Play and at What Level

In the *Journal of Bone and Joint Surgery,* surgeons warn: "High levels of sporting activities can be detrimental to the long-term success of hip resurfacing devices, independently from other risk factors. Patients seeking hip resurfacing are usually young and should limit their involvement in sports to levels that the implant construct will be able to tolerate."[179]

What is the Difference Between Hip Resurfacing and Hip Replacement?

Hip resurfacing is not hip replacement. In hip resurfacing the head of the femur is capped (after being trimmed) with a smooth metal covering. The damaged bone and cartilage within the socket is removed and replaced with a metal cup, similar to that in a total hip replacement.

In total hip replacement, not only is the head of the femur replaced, but also the socket in the pelvis (acetabulum).

One of the main selling points for hip resurfacing is that it leaves more bone so a hip replacement can be performed later.

I see hip resurfacing as one hip surgery setting up another. Surgery in my opinion should always be the last option.

Is Hip Resurfacing Really a Less Invasive Technique?

According to surgeons, hip resurfacing is more difficult to perform and requires a larger incision than typical hip replacement. This increases the risk of complications.

For an athlete or a worker whose profession is physically demanding, or any other patient, this can mean unexpected down time and costs.

Does Hip Resurfacing Keep a Younger Patient Active?

Another main selling feature for hip resurfacing as opposed to hip replacement is that studies have shown that it allows the patient to remain more active. However, it is for a limited amount of time. Hip resurfacing has an unknown life span. Thereafter, hip replacement is often necessary.

There can be more issues in relation to the soft tissue needed to stabilize the hip:

Doctors in the medical journal *Radiographics* suggest: "Surgical management for hip disorders should preserve the soft tissue constraints in the hip when possible to maintain normal hip biomechanics."[180]

This is exactly why we see so many patients after hip surgery. It is too often that the soft tissue that holds the tendons to the bone, or the ligaments that hold the bones to the bones, are compromised.

Strengthened ligaments and tendons help hold the hip joint in its proper place, causing less grinding and less bone-on-bone. Restored collagen can help rebuild the cartilage between the pelvis and thighbone, cushioning and relieving the bone-on-bone condition. This is when a consultation for Stem Cell Therapy and Platelet-Rich Plasma

Therapy should be considered—and hopefully prior to rather than after surgery: once a prosthesis has been implanted, it is too late to regenerate tissue.

More Hip Problems that May Confuse the Diagnosis

PIRIFORMIS SYNDROME

Piriformis syndrome may cause pain in the buttocks, lower back, or down the leg. The piriformis muscle is in the buttocks, attaches to the pelvis and greater trochanter, and helps rotate the leg outward. The sciatic nerve is just beneath it. Occasionally the nerve is impinged beneath the piriformis muscle. When the muscle contracts, it pushes on the nerve, which causes the pain and its radiation down the leg. I rarely see true piriformis syndrome. Typically, the pain is at the enthesis of the piriformis or other buttocks muscles to the bone, and PRP usually heals that with one to three treatments.

GREATER TROCHANTERIC BURSITIS AND ISCHIAL BURSITIS

The areas around the hip are covered with and protected by several bursal fluid filled sacs. Each bursa produces lubricating fluid and functions to reduce pressure and friction around the muscles and ligaments over bone. These bursae can become irritated from injury, excessive pressure, and overuse. Inflammation of a bursa is called bursitis. More often this diagnosis is actually a tendinitis or tendinosis. Nevertheless, PRP is usually the correct treatment. Certainly not steroids, like cortisone, which deteriorate the tissue, and can make it worse later.

HIP EFFUSION

There is normally a small amount of synovial fluid contained in the hip joint that allows the cartilage on the bones to slide on each other. An excess of this fluid, often caused by overuse or arthritis, can cause pressure and pain in the joint. The fluid comes from synovial tissue surrounding the joint.

I use an ultrasound to visualize the joint, and if an effusion is present, I numb the area and aspirate the fluid. At the same time, platelet-rich plasma or stem cells can be injected through the same needle. Effusions are removed to reduce the joint pressure and to eliminate dilution of the regenerating cells from the patient's body.

HIP TENDINITIS OR TEARS

Tendinitis occurs when a muscle is overused and pulls on the tendon that attaches it to the bone. In the hip, tendons perform an important role by keeping strong muscles attached to the femur (thighbone) as the legs move. One kind of tendinitis that occurs as a result of overuse is called iliacus tendinitis or iliopsoas tendinitis. The iliac muscle, which starts at the hip bone, and the psoas muscle, which starts in your lower spine, are used when lifting the leg toward the chest. They come together in a tendon at the top of the femur, and that is the point where tendinitis occurs.

The problems of the hip can often be treated with Stem Cell Therapy and Platelet-Rich Plasma Therapy. In order to determine if you are a good candidate for this type of procedure, you need to be fully evaluated by a physician who has significant experience with hip pain.

TERRIBLE SIDE EFFECTS

Unfortunately, too many patients come to me after a hip replacement or other "elective" surgery. The most recent disaster is happening to a very old friend of mine. He is 65 years old, and had both hips replaced for osteoarthritis a few years ago. I previously told him not to do the surgeries and that he really didn't need them. We had dinner last week, and he told me of an "odd" situation that occurs around his surgical scars. Occasionally, the scar and surrounding tissue becomes red and swollen. None of his doctors can figure out why. Allergy to the prosthetic metal, plastic, or glue inside his body? I didn't pay much attention since it didn't sound that bad. Two nights ago, he sent me photos of a recent out-break. The area of redness and swelling was about four inches by eight inches. I told him to go directly to the

ER since it looked like an infection. He was told by the ER doc that he didn't know what to do, and that my friend should see a dermatologist. Unfortunately, no derm was available for several days in the rural area where my friend lives. I am on pins and needles waiting for the diagnosis, if anyone can figure it out. My guess is that my friend will have to have his prostheses removed and replaced with another material, with the hope that the "allergy" will not return. To me the skin looked so inflamed that if no infection was present, it certainly could occur anytime. I have not told him yet what I am thinking, and am glad this book will not be published for him to read for a couple more months.

I'm not going to implant you with terrible stories of what I have seen after surgeries on many different parts of the body. Since the time I became involved in surgery in 1989, I have seen more bad outcomes than I care to remember. And let me make it clear that I respect surgeons for the difficult and complex work that they do. To me, they are the masters of medicine. Not many of us are willing to bear such standards and responsibilities. However, I must say that in my humble opinion, most elective surgeries should not be done. The risks are just too high.

7

Shoulder Pain

The shoulder is a common source of disability, often resulting from traumatic and degenerate tears of the rotator cuff or labrum, subacromial bursitis, impingement, and osteoarthritis. Nonoperative management has too often focused on narcotics, other analgesics, anti-inflammatory medications, and steroid injections such as cortisone.

The proper diagnosis of shoulder pain is essential in order to determine the root cause of the problem and the proper method of treatment. Because many shoulder conditions are caused by specific activities, a detailed medical history is an invaluable tool. A physical examination should also include screening for physical abnormalities, including swelling, deformity, muscle weakness, and tender areas, along with the range of shoulder motion.

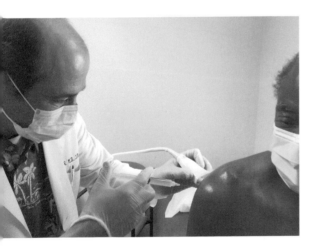

Shoulder Surgery Failures

Despite research showing surgical failures, more patients are having shoulder replacement surgery. The most common indications for shoulder arthroplasty (replacement) are osteoarthritis, inflammatory arthritis, proximal humerus fracture, irreparable rotator cuff tear, rotator cuff arthropathy, and avascular necrosis of the humeral head. In one study, radiologists looked for key imaging features of these indications. These features facilitate a correlative understanding between the initial diagnosis and the choice of type of arthroplasty used. These include total shoulder arthroplasty,[181] which is acceptable if surgery is the only option. For many patients, however, surgery can be avoided.

In a recent study, doctors discuss hardware failures known to plague patients: "The longevity of total shoulder replacement is primarily limited by the performance of the ultra high-molecular-weight polyethylene glenoid component. [This study] demonstrates that glenoid component fracture associated with oxidation has not been eliminated with the advent of modern materials (HXL) in the shoulder domain." In other words, a hardware problem not fixed.[182]

Another problem with shoulder replacement is bone disintegration—an issue that Stem Cell Therapy has been shown to heal.

From one research study: "Subchondral bone changes associated with osteoarthritis may be important factors to consider when choosing a replacement component. For surgical treatment, many implant options exist, and survivability is often dependent on patient age, activity level, and progression of osteoarthritis."[183]

If bone must be repaired in preparation for surgery, why not repair the bone to avoid surgery? The shoulder is a difficult joint to replace, and a failed shoulder replacement is even more difficult to replace.

The following research from the *Journal of Shoulder and Elbow Surgery* explains why patients must be given information on treatment options outside of surgery: "The management of a failed shoulder represents a complex and difficult problem for the treating surgeon, with potential difficulties and complications that are related to the need to remove a well-fixed stem."[184] If the prosthesis is removed due to failure, the bone becomes compromised, and it is even more difficult to place another prosthesis.

Doctors are looking for shoulder replacement alternatives. One study found that surgical repairs of degenerate and torn tissue are often prone to failure, and that some biological (biomedical) therapies (such as Platelet-Rich Plasma Therapy or Stem Cell Therapy) might improve outcomes. In fact, injections of platelet-rich plasma have led to reduced pain and improved recovery in other degenerated areas, together with the restoration of function.[185]

Doctors in Germany looked at repairing cartilage defects and soft tissue injury in the shoulder before it leads to advanced osteoarthritis. They concluded that Stem Cell Therapy for cartilage regeneration was a minimally invasive approach for shoulder joint preservation and an alternative to shoulder replacement.[186]

A proper diagnosis of the shoulder pain is essential to determine the root cause of the problem and the best method of treatment, research suggests: "Clinical decision-making is made more difficult because of the variable presentations observed in patients with a documented full-thickness rotator cuff tear: some have good function and no pain, some have good function and pain, some have poor function and no pain, and some have both poor function and pain."[187]

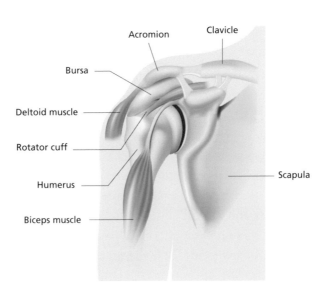

Acromion

Clavicle

Bursa

Deltoid muscle

Rotator cuff

Humerus

Biceps muscle

Scapula

Because it is difficult to determine what the pain generator is, my approach is to regenerate the entire shoulder, including, but not limited to the rotator cuff tendons, the glenoid and acromioclavicular joints, the labrum, ligaments, and the subdeltoid bursa.

In the worst case of shoulder replacement I have seen, an elderly man presented with right shoulder pain. When I asked him to lift his arms, he lifted his right arm, but had no motion at all in his left shoulder. I was perplexed and asked if his left shoulder also hurt. His response was alarming. He told me that he had a left shoulder replacement, and the arm prosthesis had dislocated out of the shoulder, and he had absolutely no use of his left arm since the dislocation that could not be relocated into the false joint. He obviously wanted to avoid surgery to his right shoulder.

Rotator Cuff Tear Treatments

Researchers say that despite increasing medical knowledge, treating shoulder pain—whether in workers, the aging, athletes, or others—remains one of the most challenging tasks in medicine. The problem? Continued shoulder tearing and degeneration after treatment.

Researchers looked at the long-term risks of rotator cuff tear enlargement and symptom progression associated with degenerative asymptomatic tears. They collected patients who had tears but no symptoms in one shoulder, and pain due to rotator cuff disease in the other shoulder. Among the 224 patients in the study, who were followed for an average of five years, there were:

- 118 initial full-thickness tears
- 56 initial partial-thickness tears
- 50 undiagnosed controls

Results:

- Tear enlargement was seen in 49% of the shoulders within an average of 2.8 years.
- Of the 244 subjects, 100 (46%) developed new pain.[188]

According to a study on athletes, "The results of treatment are not as predictable as the patient, family, trainer, coach, and doctor would like to think."[189]

Effectiveness of Rotator Cuff Tear Surgery

There has long been a debate over the effectiveness of rotator cuff tear surgery. Numerous medical studies have shown that the re-tear rate of a surgically repaired shoulder can be anywhere from 20% to 90%, depending on the patient's particular circumstances. Australian researchers presenting at the American Academy of Orthopaedic Surgeons (AAOS) 2012 Annual Meeting said that the failure rate they measured among 500 patients was 57%.

I see many patients in my office who have had a shoulder surgery with less than expected results. Worsening complications may include infection, increased stiffness, weakness, instability, decreased range of motion, and, of course, increased pain.

Now doctors are trying to answer surgical concerns postoperatively with growth factors of regenerative medicine, namely Platelet-Rich Plasma Therapy (PRP) and Stem Cell Therapy. Recent research notes that the goal of rotator cuff surgery is return of strength, mechanical stability, and healing of the tendon-to-bone interface. Advances in the understanding of rotator cuff biology and biomechanics, as well as improvements in surgical techniques, have led to the development of new strategies that may allow a tendon-to-bone interface healing process rather than the formation of fibrovascular scar tissue. Such strategies involve the use of PRP, stem cells, and other growth factors.

Stem Cell Therapy, Platelet-Rich Plasma Therapy, and Prolotherapy for Rotator Cuff Injury

If surgeons are eager to use PRP and stem cells in wound healing after surgery, why not be as eager to try it before the surgery?

Most recently, doctors in Switzerland compared PRP injections to cortisone injections in the shoulder. The doctors found good results

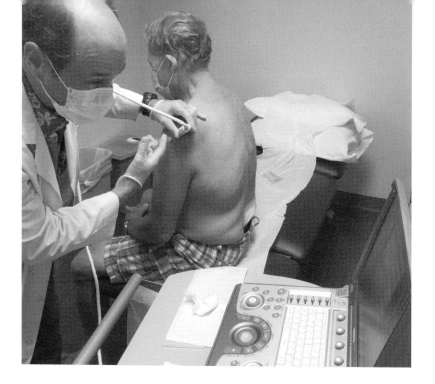

for the PRP and were able to conclude that PRP injections are a good alternative to cortisone injections, especially in patients with contraindication to cortisone.[190] Similarly, other research has suggested that bone marrow Stem Cell Therapy showed encouraging results in pain and motion relief for patients with rotator cuff and shoulder osteoarthritis.[191]

SLAP Lesions (Superior Labral Anterior Posterior)

The surgical treatment of labral (tissue around shoulder joint) SLAP tears continues to be challenging for both physicians and patients. Of course, it becomes much more challenging to the patient if the surgery does not work to the patient's expectations. A 2016 paper stated that tears of the superior labrum involving the biceps anchor are a common occurrence, especially in athletes, and may highly impair shoulder function. If conservative treatment fails, successful arthroscopic repair of symptomatic SLAP lesions has been described in the literature, particularly for young athletes.

However, the results for athletes whose sport involves throwing are less successful, with a significant proportion of patients who will not regain their pre-injury level of performance.

The clinical results of SLAP repairs in middle-aged and older patients are mixed, with worse results and higher revision rates compared to younger patients. In this population, tenotomy (surgical division of a tendon) or tenodesis (suturing of the end of the biceps tendon to the bone) are viable alternatives to SLAP repairs in order to improve clinical outcomes.[192] In tenodesis, the surgeon moves the bicep tendon attachment to a different place on the bone (usually as part of a more complex surgery).

SLAP (Labral) Lesions May Actually be Rare Injuries

Recently, Dr. Stephen C. Weber presented the findings of his study showing that American Board of Orthopaedic Surgery (ABOS) Part II candidates (young surgeons) may be performing superior labral tear anterior to posterior (SLAP) repairs at greater rates than they should. He noted that the increase in surgeries was leading to poor outcomes and increased complication rates.

One of the reasons too many surgeries were being performed was because MRI suggested a SLAP tear when SLAP tears were not there. Dr. Weber noted that magnetic resonance imaging (MRI) scans often produce false positives and that SLAP lesions are difficult to diagnose clinically. Numerous studies suggest that even experts disagree on how to define a type II SLAP tear.

"Furthermore, repairing SLAPs is not a benign process, and caring for failed SLAPs can be very difficult," said Dr. Weber. "Complications include stiffness, persistent rotator cuff tears next to the portals, and damage to the articular cartilage." He expressed particular concern about the number of older patients receiving SLAP tear repairs because of the potential for a significant number of complications and poor outcomes.

Dr. Weber suggested that educating young orthopaedists to distinguish between pathologic SLAP lesions and incidental degeneration of the labrum might help to reduce the rates of SLAP repair and improve outcomes. "I think we need to do a better job of defining labral pathology for the patients who truly have symptomatic SLAP lesions," he said.[193]

Too many times I see patients complaining of continued pain after a failed labral repair. Was the "torn" labrum the pain generator? Probably not, or perhaps the surgery may have caused more damage. Consider what happens when a knife cuts into the body and tools are used to "repair" the area. And why is it that I often see patients with pain and loss of range of motion that show no pathology on MRI. I am pressing you to understand that as doctors we really don't always know exactly what is going on, even after the history, physical, and diagnostic films. That's why my first law of medicine is to be conservative, and do no harm. And with this in mind in light of too many surgeries being done, *why not regenerate the tissue instead of cutting it out?*

Is shoulder surgery the answer for the athlete who wants a quick return to their sport? For many athletes and non-athletes, the answer is yes, because the alternative recommendations from their orthopedic specialist of ice, rest, physical therapy and waiting six months is not the option they want. And honestly, even today, most surgeons—even those who do PRP and Stem Cells—do not believe alternative therapies work, using them simply as a way to bring patients into the office. When the pain persists after an incomplete course of treatment, surgery is then recommended.

Unfortunately, the process of tissue regrowth often takes several treatments over several weeks. I always suggest nonsurgical options, since, as noted at the start of this book, I personally had a failed shoulder surgery that made my shoulder much worse. After surgery, my arm filled with fluid, I had a fever, and large blisters developed on my arm and shoulder. I liked my surgeon, who was my professor while I was doing orthopedic surgery in my training—but at that point I realized that surgery was a mistake in many instances, and I questioned whether I still wanted to make it my lifetime work. When I learned about regenerative medicine, I injected my own shoulder and the pain was gone when I awakened the next morning. My shoulder remained pain-free for twelve years until I reinjured it, at which point I repeated the injections, and again healed my own shoulder. It has been pain-free since then.

Shoulder Impingement: Surgery Not Often the Answer

Researchers state that surgical interventions for subacromial impingement syndrome do not reveal one surgical technique to be better than another, nor do they show that surgery is superior in any way to conservative interventions.[194]

Further data shows, when young athletes have arthroscopic stabilization surgery, it must be emphasized to the patients and their families that the recurrence rate following arthroscopic procedures is higher in young people than in the adult population.[195]

Shoulder impingement surgery may not be the fastest way back to health. A patient with problems of the rotator cuff or shoulder impingement may think that surgery will be a quick fix. However, surgery is an invasive procedure that often requires lengthy recovery and physical therapy *even* if it is successful. Further, even "successful" surgery may not relieve the pain, and shoulder weakness can remain. Complications can also include nerve damage and increased weakness.

One study noted that "[m]ost patients experience pain relief and functional improvement following arthroscopic rotator cuff repair, but some continue to experience symptoms post-operatively. Patients with so-called failed rotator cuff syndrome, that is, with continued pain, weakness, and limited active range of motion following arthroscopic rotator cuff repair, present a diagnostic and therapeutic challenge."[196]

The traditional treatment options include another surgery to repair the first one, or surgery to transfer a tendon into the area, and arthroplasty.

Shoulder Impingement Surgery Alternatives

Although "impingement" refers specifically to pressure on the tendons and bursa in the shoulder, it is a generalized term often used to refer to shoulder pain of unknown origin. Other terms used are tendinitis, tendinosis, and bursitis, when none of these are actually proven as pain generators.

Stem Cell Therapy, Platelet-Rich Plasma (PRP) Therapy, and Prolotherapy are injection techniques that can accelerate the body's own regenerative actions to repair the worn or injured tissue.

By isolating the areas that are damaged and injecting these spots with various "proliferants"—which may range from hypoertonic dextrose (Prolotherapy) to your own blood platelets or stem cells—the practitioner is summoning the natural injury-repair mechanism of the body to the area that needs healing. Part of the cure is the manufactured, controlled inflammation caused by these proliferants. This stimulates a new collagen matrix, which makes the tissue stronger and thicker and can restore it to its pain-free state.

In a recent study, doctors found that following Prolotherapy treatments, patients with refractory chronic rotator cuff disease showed improvement in the areas of pain, disability, isometric strength, and range of motion.[197]

Most recently, doctors in Switzerland compared PRP injections to cortisone in the shoulder. The doctors found good results for the PRP and were able to conclude that PRP injections are a good alternative to cortisone injections, especially in patients with contraindication to cortisone.[198]

There are many injuries that result in 100% tearing of the rotator cuff tendons in previously healthy shoulders. These often occur in sports, car accidents, or situations where the shoulder is exposed to sudden extreme force.

Even with complete tendon tear, Stem Cell Therapy, PRP, and Prolotherapy, may be the preferred treatment. Occasionally, surgery to repair torn tissue might be the only option. Even so, Stem Cell Therapy and PRP can accelerate healing after surgery.

Shoulder Dislocation

The shoulder comprises a complex matrix of bone and soft tissue that enables an extreme range of motion. But the price the shoulder pays for that range of motion is a greater risk of chronic injury.

Shoulder Dislocation

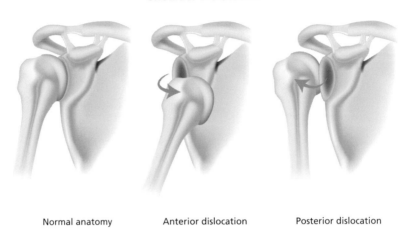

Normal anatomy   Anterior dislocation   Posterior dislocation

The shoulder is held together by soft tissue stabilizers, the ligaments that connect bone to bone. Over the course of time, especially in sports that involve heavy shoulder-to-shoulder contact (such as hockey, lacrosse, football, wrestling, and basketball), the ligaments may stretch out and become "lax." When the ligaments become lax, the risk of dislocation and separation becomes greater.

In a study published in the *British Journal of Sports Medicine*, researchers took a look at rugby players with measurable shoulder laxity to gauge the risk of shoulder dislocation. What they found was that 50% of the athletes tested were at significant risk.

It is estimated that 95% of shoulder dislocations occur when athletes suffer a blow to the shoulder that forces the shoulder joint "back" or downward, or occur when they fall to the ground with their arms stretched over their heads.

Chronic Shoulder Dislocation Treatment

Traumatic shoulder dislocation is a frequent injury in the sports population. An acute shoulder dislocation often means a one-time traumatic episode, whereas chronic shoulder instability indicates multiple recurrent dislocations.

Following an initial shoulder dislocation, doctors debate whether or not to perform surgery to prevent recurrence. If there is an accompanying labral or tendon tear, that can be addressed along with tightening of the capsule around the joint. This can lead to a loss of range of motion. I have used Stem Cell Therapy with platelets (both are in the bone marrow) or just PRP from the blood, both with good results, to tighten the shoulder after a failed surgery for chronic dislocations.

If the patient is under 30 years of age, shoulder surgery is typically recommended by surgeons because younger athletes are much more prone to repeated dislocations than older athletes.

Until recently, it was common in cases of dislocation to immobilize the shoulder for long periods of time. But studies showed that while immobilization helped alleviate the pain of such injuries, it also contributed to a general weakening of the ligaments and predominance of "adhesive capsulitis," where the arm is frozen (frozen shoulder) and can no longer be lifted.

Surgery for shoulder dislocation can be effective for some but, as always, surgery should be considered a last option because of issues of complications, downtime (immobilization), and—for both the "weekend warrior" and the professional athlete—a weakening of the shoulder through the removal of or damage to other connective tissue in the surgical process.

Some athletes may opt for immediate surgery because of the typical six-month healing time (if healing occurs at all) required in the case of a Bankart lesion (an injury of the anterior [inferior] glenoid labrum) without Stem Cell Therapy or PRP. Researchers have pointed out that "[r]epairs of degenerate and torn tissue are often prone to failure due to many intrinsic and extrinsic factors" and that Platelet-Rich Plasma Therapy has been shown to reduce pain and improve recovery in shoulder tears.[199]

The key to avoiding shoulder surgery or shoulder separation requiring surgery is to strengthen the shoulder girdle. This can be accomplished by working the strong shoulder muscle group and by treating the weakened shoulder ligaments with injections of regenerative medicine.

To understand the importance of having strong ligaments to hold the shoulder together, the patient needs to understand that the severity of the shoulder dislocation is measured by the degree of injury to the ligaments and the amount of instability of the joint.

Shoulder Separation

The acromioclavicular (AC) and the coracoclavicular (CC) ligaments hold the shoulder together at the point where the collarbone (clavicle) and the top (acromion) of the shoulder meet. This joint can also be traumatically separated. I see this most commonly in bicycling accidents in which the patient has flown over the handlebars and landed on the shoulder.

This is a very small joint that heals well with regenerative medicine.

- In type I level separation, the AC is partially torn; the CC is not.
- In type II separation, the AC is completely torn; the CC is partially or not torn.
- In type III separation, both ligaments are completely torn.

With this injury one can often see the collarbone sticking up above the top of the shoulder. Obviously, the more significant the tearing, the longer the athlete is out of their sport.

Untreated shoulder instability can lead to an alteration of an athlete's game to protect the sore shoulder, or, worse, chronic shoulder separation that can keep athletes away from their sport for significant amounts of time.

Stem Cell Therapy and PRP use the patient's own cells to repair and rebuild ligaments and the joint itself.

8

Other Conditions

Elbow

There is some new and exciting research to share on elbow pain and instability.

Tennis elbow (lateral epicondylitis) is a term for elbow tendinitis, an inflammation, soreness, or pain on the outside (lateral) part of the upper arm near the elbow. The cause is usually common extensor tendinosis or a partial tear in the tendon fibers, which connect muscle to the bone. The traditional term tendinitis refers to the acute (recent) inflammatory stage of tendon injury, while the new term, tendinosis refers to the chronic injury when inflammatory cells are no longer seen, but the tendon is worn.

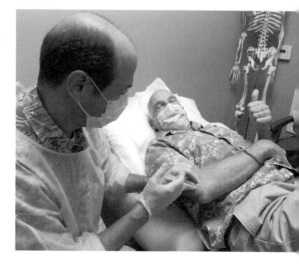

Symptoms include elbow pain that gradually worsens and can radiate outside of the elbow to the forearm and the back of the hand.

Although termed "tennis elbow," anyone can experience this painful condition that results from overuse of the tendon, such as in keyboarding.

Patients with tennis elbow may not respond to the conventional treatments of "wait, rest, and medicate for pain relief." For many patients, this slow track to healing is not on their schedule. Most patients prefer getting on with their lives by fast-forwarding the healing process.

PRP for Tennis Elbow

Platelet-Rich Plasma Therapy extracts the healing platelets from the patient's blood and then re-injects the platelet-rich plasma into the injured elbow tendon. I find that injecting the joint at the same time also speeds healing.

In a comparison of PRP and cortisone injections, doctors found PRP to be a superior treatment option over the long term.[200]

In another comparison study, doctors examined treatment with autologous blood injections verses painkillers, cortisone, and PRP. Of these three options, PRP injections were found to improve pain with a lower risk of complications.[201]

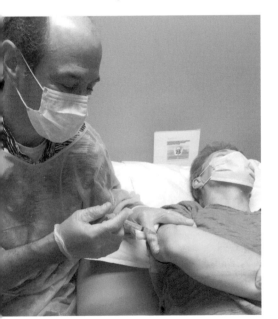

Recent research in the *American Journal of Sports Medicine* documented the positive effects of PRP on tennis elbow. Patients treated with PRP had significantly less pain and greater function, exceeding the effect of corticosteroid injection, even after a follow-up of two years.[202]

Research in the *British Journal of Sports Medicine* states that cortisone should never be used, and that injection therapies such as

PRP and simple dextrose Prolotherapy can be effective and excellent treatments for tennis elbow.[203]

In addition, research published in the *Journal of Hand and Microsurgery* examined the effectiveness of PRP injections. It was found that PRP injections have an important and effective role in the treatment of elbow instability.[204]

In the journal *BioMed Research International*, doctors reviewing the medical literature found that the first studies on Stem Cell Therapy showed promising results for elbow pain.

That same research showed that patients who had received a series of three separate Prolotherapy injections over a period of 8 weeks had significantly improved pain scores and isometric strength at 16 weeks compared to a placebo.[205]

In several failed cases I have seen, surgical removal of the extensor tenson from the bone was performed, and resutured to the bone. I honestly am not sure why this procedure is ever done. These patients present to me with a prominant scar. In all cases to date, regenerative medicine completed the cure.

Neck and Cervical Spine

I regularly see patients who have been told by another doctor that they need surgery for neck instability, or who have already had a failed cervical spine surgery.

Why do so many patients undergo neck surgery? One reason is their fear that symptoms may progress. Another is that they are sometimes told they may be risking paralysis without it. Most commonly, though, it is because the doctor does not know how to heal neck pain due to ligament injury.

Is "Unstable" Spondylolisthesis Really Unstable?

For many patients with "unstable" cervical degenerative spondylolisthesis, observation may be a better choice than surgery, according to the researchers who conducted a study described below.

Degenerative spondylolisthesis refers to a slipped vertebrae caused by vertebral fracture or attenuation of the *pars inarticularis*, a part of the vertebra. Because spondylolisthesis is commonly thought to result in instability of the cervical spine, spinal fusion surgery (arthrodesis) is sometimes considered the appropriate treatment. The authors of this study wrote: "Our results suggest that the majority of these patients may be stable and do not develop progression of disease or catastrophic neurologic deficits."

The researchers analyzed the natural history of cervical degenerative spondylolisthesis in 27 patients.

The 16 men and 11 women in the study underwent cervical spine radiographs (x-rays) on two occasions at least two years apart. The patients' average age at the time of the initial radiograph was 59 years; average time to the follow-up radiographs was 39 months. Measurements on the paired radiographs were carefully compared to determine whether and how much the cervical slippage increased over time.

Initial x-rays showed instability (at least two millimeters of displacement between vertebrae) in several patients. However, during follow-up, none of the patients showed further progression, defined as additional displacement of two millimeters or more. The average progression was only about one-half millimeter.

Twenty-one patients had backward displacement (retrolisthesis) of the cervical vertebrae, while six had forward displacement (anterolisthesis). The patients with retrolisthesis had somewhat greater slippage during follow-up; however, none had a dislocation or suffered neurological damage.

No Progression of Slippage or Symptoms

Of 16 patients who had symptoms such as neck pain or sensory abnormalities at the initial visit, most were successfully managed without surgery. Of the 11 patients who were initially symptom-free, none developed symptoms during follow-up.

The study is one of the few to look at the natural history of the results and suggests that at medium-term follow-up, the conditions appear to be "relatively stable" in most patients. Dr. Park and colleagues write: "This begs the question, if an 'unstable' spine does fine without treatment, is it really unstable?

Our results suggest that the majority of these patients may be stable and do not develop progression of disease or catastrophic neurologic deficits."

The researchers acknowledge some important limitations of their study—particularly the small number of patients and relatively short follow-up period. However, the results suggest that for many patients, cervical spondylolisthesis is a nonprogressive condition that does not necessarily require surgical treatment. The authors conclude, "In the absence of neurologic symptoms, we recommend observation of patients with degenerative spondylolistheses of the cervical spine."[206]

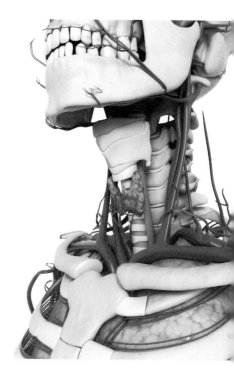

Doctors suggest in the medical journal Spine: "With many surgeons expanding their indications for cervical spine surgery, the number of patients being treated operatively has increased. Unfortunately, the number of patients requiring revision procedures is also increasing, but very little literature exists reviewing changes in the indications or operative planning for revision reconstruction."[207]

Compounding this is the ever-present rush to surgery spurred on by MRI: "Physicians should be aware of inconsistencies inherent in the interpretation of cervical MRI findings and should be aware that some findings demonstrate lower agreement than others."[208]

Neck pain is one of the problems we commonly see in my office. There are a number of ways to incur a neck injury, which damages the tendons and ligaments around the joints of the neck. Alternative symptoms associated with this type of damage can include headaches, jaw pain, ear pain, vertigo, loss of voice or hoarseness, and even irritable bowel syndrome. Some of the symptoms can often be alleviated with Stem Cell Therapy, PRP, or Prolotherapy.

One study noted successful Prolotherapy injections in traumatic cervical instability, and suggested that this type of treatment should be explored as a viable option to cervical fusion surgery.[209]

Whiplash

Hyperextension neck injuries, more commonly referred to as whiplash, are a complex problem for patients. In one study, doctors found that individuals with whiplash-associated disorders reported more additional causes of pain, more painful locations, and higher pain intensity than individuals with chronic neck pain from other causes.[210]

Patients with whiplash-related disorders also have a greater fear of movement, and doctors are calling for revising standardized tests to determine the extent of the patients' problems.[211]

Further, doctors are seeking reasons why some people recover within months and others report symptoms for extended periods. They find a strong and plausible association, as does the study above, between severe disability, clinical levels of pain, catastrophizing, and low mental health.[212]

Temporomandibular Joint Pain (TMJ)

The temporomandibular joint (TMJ) is located where the jawbone meets the cranium (the part of the skull that holds the brain). The condition known as temporomandibular joint syndrome develops from a combination of interrelated factors, usually starting with poor head posture, that contribute to the stretching and weakening of the cervical ligaments and lateral TMJ ligaments. As a result, the lower jaw can slip forward, aggravating the situation further by putting additional stress on the ligaments and the joints.

One characteristic of TMJ is the loud popping or clicking of bones rubbing together in the loosened joint, accompanied by pain and stiffness as the muscles tighten, compensating for the ligament laxity.

Conventional treatments include TMJ arthroscopy and various types of surgery, TMJ implants, injections of botulinum toxins, and cauterization. All of these treatments are invasive and somewhat risky, and their use as the chosen treatment for TMJ may ignore or even cause negative consequences.

New evidence is emerging that Platelet-Rich Plasma (PRP) Therapy might be of assistance in the treatment of degenerative conditions of the joints.

In the first study done on this, doctors in Egypt studied 50 patients with TMJ-osteoarthritis. They found that PRP performed better than hyaluronic acid injections during long-term follow-up in terms of pain reduction and increased interincisal distance (i.e., the ability to open the mouth widely).[213]

Doctors in Turkey concluded that patients suffering from TMJ disc dislocation benefited more from PRP injections than from surgery to manipulate the jaw back into place. Clearly, PRP stabilized the joint and reduced chronic instability.[214]

Doctors in Poland found that platelet-rich plasma injections into the temporomandibular joints have a positive impact on the reduction of the intensity of pain experienced by patients being treated for temporomandibular joint dysfunction.[215]

The above research does not surprise Prolotherapy practitioners, who have used regenerative medicine for years as a way to rebuild the soft tissue and the TMJ. This was confirmed in research: "Prolotherapy with 10% dextrose appears promising for the treatment of symptomatic TMJ hypermobility, as evidenced by the therapeutic benefits, simplicity, safety, patients' acceptance of the injection technique, and lack of significant side effects."[216] Even more effective than dextrose injections are PRP and stem cell therapy.

Tendons

Tendons are the small, strong, thick bands of connective tissue that connect muscles to bone.

I frequently see patients who have had an MRI of a tendon tear or chronic tendinopathy. "Tendinopathy" is a relatively recent term that is used to describe the pathology of a tendon that causes pain. The condition has classical symptoms of tenderness on palpation, as well as pain when exercising or with movement. Tendinopathy is divided into two broad categories:

Tendinitis is typically the result of a new injury, and is present during the early phase when the injury is causing inflammation—a sign that the body is trying to heal the tendon.

Tendinosis occurs at a later stage, when the tendon shows wear but no inflammation. The absence of inflammation is often due to the use of anti-inflammatory medications, which block the regeneration of collagen, the major constituent of the tendon. Yes, inflammation is needed for healing.

Most tendon injuries we see are from athletes and those who do fitness and weight training. But even an inactive person can twist an ankle or move any joint improperly, stretching and straining a tendon. The place where a tendon, ligament, or muscle attaches to bone is called the enthesis, and if the strain (tendon or muscle injury) or sprain (ligament injury) occurs at that junction with the bone, it is called an enthesopathy. Regenerative medicine is the best way I know to heal that.

Anti-inflammatory drugs and cortisone injections are effective at reducing pain and inflammation, but do not have a healing effect. In fact, their use can result in a nonhealing tendon or ligament. Further, they may lead to complete rupture, which may require surgical repair.

In the latest research, doctors who have conducted animal studies have suggested that bone-marrow derived stem cells accelerate tendon healing.[217] In published research, inverstigators announced: "Tendon injuries represent, even today, a challenge, as repair may be exceedingly slow and incomplete. Regenerative medicine and stem cell technology have shown to be of great promise."[218]

Most recently, studies have indicated the potential effectiveness of bone marrow (stem cells and platelets) and its positive effects on Achilles tendon healing, particularly during the early phases.[219]

Patellar tendinopathy is a condition that has been shown to respond very favorably to the regenerative technique of PRP. Researchers in the Netherlands report: "After PRP treatment, patients with patellar tendinopathy showed a statistically significant improvement. In addition, these improvements can also be considered clinically meaningful."[220]

Shoulder Tendons

Doctors in Switzerland recently compared PRP injections with cortisone injections in the shoulder. They found good results for PRP and were able to conclude that PRP injections are a valuable alternative to cortisone injections, especially in patients with contraindications to cortisone.[221] Other recent research suggested that bone marrow Stem Cell Therapy produced encouraging results in pain and motion relief for patients with rotator cuff and shoulder osteoarthritis.[222]

Tendinopathies

Doctors have looked at the increasing popularity of Platelet-Rich Plasma Therapy for soft tissue injuries such as ligament, muscle, tendon tears and tendinopathies.

In Achilles tendinopathy and plantar fasciitis, PRP is an effective and safe alternative for the management of patients with a poor response to conventional nonsurgical treatment.[223]

A second study confirmed the findings: "Non-insertional Achilles tendinopathy commonly impedes the functioning of active persons. Treatment methods vary, as do their results. [In this study] PRP was injected into the affected Achilles tendon of 14 prospectively selected patients [15 Achilles tendons]. . . . During follow-up, a significant improvement was observed in the clinical and imaging results."[224] A third study from September 2015 evaluated the positive long-term clinical outcomes in patients affected by mid-portion Chronic Recalcitrant Achilles Tendinopathies who received a single PRP treatment.[225]

In tendinosis and tendinitis, tears to the Achilles tendon may be caused by two different conditions. Tendinosis shows no inflammation, and no healing. It represents wearing of the tendon that may have had previous inflammation. Tendinitis shows inflammation, as the body is still trying to heal the tendon. In an attempt to stabilize the tendon, the body may deposit calcium (a condition known as calcific tendinitis, or tendinosis).

If we can create sufficient inflammation in the areas of the tendon that are damaged or worn, the tendon can often be healed, as mentioned in the research above. PRP, Stem Cell Therapy, and Prolotherapy create this often needed inflammation.

9

The Impact of Diet and Pain Medication

Fat Accumulation and Obesity Destroy Joints

"(Doctors) should take possible weight reduction into account for the treatment of knee osteoarthritis whenever a patient is significantly overweight." [226]

British Medical Journal

Researchers warn that a high-fat, high-sucrose (HFS) diet creates obesity and leads to osteoarthritis.[227]

Is it simply extra weight causing problems for the weight-bearing joints like knees, hips, and ankles? Or is it chronic inflammation? A combined team of European researchers examined not only the well-known relationship between being overweight and the weight load burden on osteoarthritic symptoms and severity, but also the possibility that accumulation of belly fat causes osteoarthritis in *non-weight bearing joints* through inflammation. Several studies suggest that overweight people are more inclined to develop osteoarthritis than people of normal weight.

Researchers suggest a possible link between osteoarthritis and obesity due to inflammatory systemic effects, which would explain the presence of symptomatic hand osteoarthritis. Even though the hand is not a weight-bearing joint, the researchers suggest that *inflammation from fat accumulation attacks joints* of any type.

The researchers observed that the onset of osteoarthritis and its symptoms may be prevented more by the loss of body fat than by weight loss.[228]

This observation may be borne out by research suggesting that adding calories from proteins to one's diet, which will lead to a shift from fat to muscle in the body, can alleviate osteoarthritis symptoms.

Research published in the *Journal of the American Medical Association* looked at three groups of test subjects who were divided into "low" protein, "middle" protein, and "high" protein diets. All the participants were given 1,000 more calories than they burned each day, with the intention of measuring the weight gain.

Here are the highlights of that study:

1. In the low-protein diet test subjects, 90 percent of the extra calories turned into body fat with a decrease of 1.5 pounds of muscle.
2. In the middle and higher-protein diet group, only 50 percent of the extra calories turned into body fat. The remainder helped account for *adding* almost 7 pounds of lean body mass (muscle).

In other words,

- less protein, *more* accumulated fat
- more protein, *less* accumulated fat, and more muscle

Further, participants on the higher-protein diets burned more calories at rest than those on the low-protein diets.[229]

It is about exercise, too. We don't want to lose muscle as we age. When we diet based on caloric restriction alone, our bodies use our muscles for protein needs, which decrease muscle size and strength. Weight loss through exercise does not decrease our muscle mass.[230]

The Effects of Pain Medication and Diet on Testosterone and Joint Pain

I see a number of patients who have advancing osteoarthritis but who are too young for joint replacement. Basically, they are being managed for joint pain until they are old enough for joint replacement. At the same time, they are losing hormones, gaining weight, and losing mobility. Typically, they have lower levels of activity, chronic pain, are becoming obese, and are on pain medications. They are, clearly, in a poor healing milieu.

An Australian research paper confirmed that low testosterone is associated with an increased risk of both knee and hip replacement in overweight and obese men. The findings suggest that low circulating sex steroids may play a role in the pathogenesis of osteoarthritis in men.[231]

In another study, doctors found that restoring testosterone levels helped aging men with their joint problems, physical activity, and quality of life.[232]

A recent study suggests that after only 30 days, patients on opioid (narcotic) medication for pain management have reduced levels of testosterone.[233]

Research has shown that opioids have a number of adverse effects, including hormonal imbalances. These imbalances have been reported to primarily involve testosterone and affect both males and females to the point of interfering with successful treatment of pain management.[234]

There is a growing body of evidence making clear that the long-term treatment of chronic pain with opioid painkiller medications puts patients at great risk for hormonal abnormalities, including lowered testosterone in both male and female patients. Lowered testosterone prevents healing and also creates other health concerns.

Testosterone is an important hormone in both women and men. Adequate levels of the hormone are required for cellular growth and repair, maintenance of muscle mass and bone, and healing.

New evidence demonstrates that opioids affect testosterone levels differently in men and women, and that severity of symptoms must be carefully weighed as symptoms manifest themselves differently.[235]

A man's joint pain may be much more severe than a woman's, despite similar problems.

Further, for some men with opioid-induced testosterone deficiency, testosterone supplementation will improve pain symptoms.[236]

Patients on a high-fat and high-carbohydrate (fructose) diet often find themselves in a nearly inescapable loop of obesity and lack of physical exercise, which contributes to low testosterone which contributes to obesity and joint pain.[237]

Fasting and Calorie Restriction for Healing

One of the most fascinating subjects in health is caloric restriction and fasting, since both have been shown to promote healing, health, and longevity.

Short-term caloric restriction suppressed oxidative stress and improved cardiac function.[238]

Caloric restriction increases the level of the hormone DHEA (short for dehydroepiandrosterone) in muscle and blood, suggesting that DHEA might partially mediate anti-aging, anti-obesity, and health-promoting effects.[239]

Caloric restriction has been found to reverse the impairment caused by a high-fat diet with very high energy efficiency in a short period.[240]

In the context of joint repair, caloric restriction becomes especially intriguing.

Caloric restriction may be beneficial for wound healing efficiency in aging individuals.[241]

In 1985, doctors at the University of Southern California released research showing that fasting triggered stem cell-based regeneration. They found that cycles of prolonged fasting not only protect against immune system damage, but also induce immune system regeneration, shifting stem cells from a dormant state to a state of self-renewal. Such findings have significant implications for healthier aging, as the decline in immune system function with aging contributes to increased susceptibility to disease. *Calorie restriction with adequate nutrition is the only nongenetic intervention, and the most consistent non-pharmacological one, that both extends the lifespan and reduces inflammation.*[242, 243]

Arthritis is related to inflammation in the joint tissue. Reducing inflammation through proper food choices and diet is something I recommend to all my patients. Then why do I use the inflammation of regenerative medicine to heal the body? Consider the following precepts:

1. Musculoskeletal pain and arthritis is often caused by chronic inflammation that is uncontrolled.
2. Regenerative medicine causes a controlled, short burst of inflammation, which is needed to initiate the growth of new tissue.
3. The short burst of inflammation brings new healing cells to the injured or worn tissue, stimulating new tissue growth which stops the chronic inflammation.

Foods that may aggravate arthritis and should be minimized in the diet:

- Foods high in saturated fat (e.g., dairy, red meat, and baked goods)
- Coffee (because of the high acid content)
- Sugary foods
- Refined grains (e.g., refined pasta, white rice, and white breads)
- Refined or processed foods (if it's in a box or a can, it's processed)
- Alcohol

Foods that help lower inflammation in the body and should be mainstays of the diet:

- Vegetables and certain fruits (create an alkaline environment)
- Whole grains, such as brown rice and bulgur wheat
- Sources of omega-3 fatty acids, such as fatty fish (e.g. salmon and mackerel), fish oil supplements, and walnuts
- Lean protein sources (e.g., chicken, turkey, or beans)
- Green tea

PRP Vampire Facelift

The same PRP healing elements that we have written about throughout this book have been successfully applied to cosmetic medicine. The utilization of Platelets and other growth factors found in your blood, trigger new collagen production. This results is tauter, smoother and more youthful skin. When combined with dermal fillers; shape, color, texture and volume are all restored with the outcome lasting approximately 18 months.

In this brief chapter we will discuss how Platelet Rich Plasma, or "The Vampire Facelift," can produce a more natural and youthful facial appearance than traditional surgical facelifts.

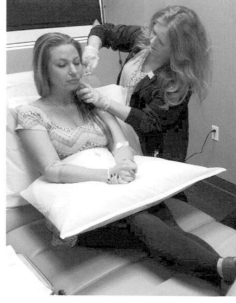

Michelle Darrow, RN, NP

Although there can be a place for a surgical facelift, such procedures are not necessarily a panacea or cure-all to the concerns of the aging face. Cosmetic surgery when needed can remove excess skin and make the person appear younger. However, a surgical facelift can actually contribute to a face collapse as the skin stretches tighter against the bone making the person look skeletonized.

What Is Vampire Face Lift?

The Vampire Facelift provides non-surgical solutions to the challenges of maintaining a youthful appearance in aging faces. The procedure addresses:

- Facial wrinkles.
- Facial volume correction such as the thinning of the dermis (volume loss) seen with weight loss.
- Improve texture of the skin and rejuvenate the complexion by using the combination of Platelet Rich Plasma therapy (PRP) and dermal fillers.
- Changes in skin color. As we age we develop dull, greying skin because of reduced blood circulation in the face. The Vampire Facelift helps restore healthy natural looking glowing skin.
- The loss of skin elasticity.
- The slow collapse of the facial structure and subsequent droopiness in the shape of the face.

The PRP used in the Vampire Facelift® is the same as that used for years at the Darrow Stem Cell Institute to effectively speed joint, tendon and tissue repair. Our extensive experience using PRP to stimulate tissue repair and regeneration combined with our vast experience injecting fillers makes the Vampire Facelift® a cinch, with impressive results!

Growth Factor Production Known Effects

1. Epidermal Growth Factor (EGF)—Stimulates fibroblasts to secrete collagenase to degrade the matrix during the remodeling phase. Stimulates keratinocyte and fibroblast proliferation.
2. Transforming Growth Factor—Promotes angiogenesis, up-regulates collagen production and inhibits degradation, promotes chemo attraction of inflammatory cells.
3. Vascular Endothelial Growth Factor (VEGF)—Endothelial cells promote angiogenesis during tissue hypoxia.

4. Fibroblast Growth Factor (FGF)—Promotes angiogenesis, granulation, and epithelialization via endothelial cell, fibroblast, and keratinocyte migration, respectively.

5. Platelet-Derived Growth Factor (PDGF)—Attracts macrophages and fibroblasts to zone of injury. Promotes collagen and proteoglycan synthesis.

6. Interleukins, Macrophages, keratinocytes, endothelial cells, lymphocytes, fibroblasts, osteoblasts, basophils, mast cells—Activates fibroblast differentiation. Induces collagen and proteoglycan synthesis.

7. Colony Stimulating Factors—Stimulates granulocyte and macrophage proliferation.

8. Keratinocyte Growth Factor—Fibroblasts stimulate keratinocyte migration, differentiation, and proliferation.

In 2002, Doctors at Yale University discussed the use of PRP following plastic surgery:

- The response of living tissue to injury is a central component in the planning of all surgical procedures.

- The wound-healing process is typically divided into three phases (inflammatory, proliferative, and remodeling) and it is a complex process where many components interact to restore a wound defect.

- Platelets and their released growth factors are pivotal in the modulation of this entire process.

- Although several techniques may be used to achieve repair after initial injury, few initiate and actually accelerate tissue regeneration. Both platelet gel and fibrin glue (body glue) are effective hemostatic agents.

- Platelet gels, unlike fibrin glue, have a high concentration of platelets that release the bioactive proteins and growth factors necessary to initiate and accelerate tissue repair and regeneration.

- In particular, two growth factors that play a major role in platelet gels are platelet-derived growth factor and transforming growth factor beta, which significantly increases and stimulates the deposition of extracellular matrix (the "soup" that cartilage grows from).

- Platelet gels have global applications in surgery and are especially useful for the soft tissue and bony reconstructions encountered in facial plastic and reconstructive surgery. In these applications, their use has been associated with a decrease in operative time, necessity for drains and pressure dressings, and incidence of complications.[244]

This study followed similar research from doctors at Florida Atlantic University who tested "PRP" gel and fibrin glue to evaluate their effectiveness in stopping capillary bleeding in the surgical flaps of patients undergoing cosmetic surgery.

The types of surgical procedures included face lifts, breast augmentations, breast reductions, and neck lifts.

Capillary bed bleeding was present in all tested cases and effectively sealed within 3 minutes following the application of platelet gel and fibrin glue.[245] Clearly, PRP is a healer and has a place in cosmetic procedures.

Reversing Sun Damage

In 2003, doctors at Scripps-XIMED Medical Center began looking at growth factors in the repair of sun damaged skin. This is what they wrote:

- Though surgical procedures may be very effective, the associated healing time and potential risks have spurred the development of non-surgical treatments.
- There has also been an increasing depth of knowledge regarding wound healing and its control by growth factors as well as its modulation by the topical application of growth factors.

The objective of this study was to determine if the twice daily application of a combination of multiple growth factors (such as those found in PRP) to photodamaged facial skin results in any evidence of improvement after 60 days.

- Eleven of 14 patients showed clinical improvement in at least one facial area. The peri-orbital (around the eyes) region showed a statistically significant improvement.
- There was a decrease in the depth and number of textural irregularities or fine lines.
- Biopsies revealed new collagen formation and thickening of the epidermis by 27%.
- Eight of 14 patients felt their wrinkles were improved, while 12 of 14 felt their skin texture was improved.

The application of a mixture of topical growth factors may stimulate the repair of facial photodamage resulting in new collagen formation, epidermal thickening and the clinical appearance of smoother skin with less visible wrinkling.[246]

Skin needling

In this study, doctors from Turkey evaluated the efficacy and safety of intradermal injection of PRP in human facial rejuvenation.

Twenty women ranging in age from 40 to 49 years were enrolled in the study. PRP increases dermal collagen levels not only by growth factors, but also by skin needling. PRP application could be considered as an effective (even a single application) and safety procedure for facial skin rejuvenation.[247]

A paper from China notes that needling can change the aging state of skin possibly by strengthening the activity of fibroblasts in the skin and by increasing the content of soluble collagen.[248]

Circulation

In a 2012 paper from the New York Eye and Ear Infirmary's department of plastic surgery. Doctors wrote how platelets created collagen, created a fat layer, and created circulation in skin. In this study:

Patients were injected with a Platelet-rich fibrin matrix in the deep dermis and immediate subdermis of the upper arms.

- Findings from examination supported the clinical observation of soft-tissue augmentation.
- As early as 7 days after treatment, activated fibroblasts (healing cells) and new collagen deposition were noted and continued to be evident throughout the 10 week course of the study.
- Development of new blood vessels was noted by 19 days; also at this time, intradermal collections of adipocytes and stimulation of subdermal adipocytes were noted (fat layers of skin).[249]

Neck revitalization

In 2010, doctors in Italy wrote in the *Journal of Drugs and Dermatology* that "Face and neck revitalization with PRP is a promising easy-to-perform technique in face and neck rejuvenation and scar attenuation." [250]

Sagging Skin

In 2014, doctors in Turkey wrote that in their patient studies, there was statistically significant difference regarding the general appearance, skin firmness-sagging and wrinkle state of the patients before and after three PRP applications.[251]

PRP Therapy Combined with Fillers (aka as Vampire Facelift®)

The original Vampire Facelift® is achievable combining the use of fillers with PRP serum. The fillers provide an instant fill or volume correction and the PRP immediately initiates a skin regeneration process. Patients can see and feel the effects immediately as their skin becomes smoother and firmer. The filler products we use in conjunction with the PRP serum are Restylane or Juvederm Ultra Plus. Both are hyaluronic acids. The use of PRP with fillers prolongs the effective filler correction for three to six months longer than when fillers are used alone.

Doctors at the University of Rome achieved positive results when PRP platelet rich plasma in combination with hyaluronic acid was used as a temporary skin substitute in aiding healing of acute and chronic open wounds of the foot and ankle.[252]

A 2016 study in the *Journal of Cosmetic Dermatology* recorded:

- A series of 94 female patients with varying degrees of facial aging signs were treated with PRP and hyaluronic acid.
- Average age was 53, youngest being 48, oldest 63. Average number of injections were about 3 and one-half.

Patients were asked to rate their personal satisfaction with their skin texture, pigmentation, and sagging. In addition, the overall results were rated by three independent physicians and the patients themselves. The outcomes were peer-reviewed, and correlations between the degree of the aesthetic scores and the number of injections were explored.

- There was a statistically significant difference in general appearance, skin firmness-sagging and skin texture according to the patients' before and after applications of PRP.
- A statistically significant correlation was found between the number of injections and overall satisfaction.[253]

PRP Therapy Used as Stand-Alone Skin Rejuvenation

Patients who don't want or need fillers can benefit from PRP to improve fine lines and improve the way their skin looks and feels. Think of PRP treatment as a NATURAL alternative to fillers. Your body is creating the corrections desired.

Areas ideal for stand-alone PRP therapy include:

- Full Face (when no filler needed)
- Neck (especially horizontal necklace lines)
- Crow's Feet
- Under the eye Fine Wrinkles
- Acne Scars

In a review study, doctors at Weill Cornell Medical College say that the vast majority of studies examined show a significant and measurable effect on cellular changes, wound healing, and facial esthetic outcomes with use of platelet preparations, both topical and injectable.[254]

In a study from Egypt, doctors took Forty-five patients with atrophic acne scars and randomly assigned to 3 equal groups:

- Group A received intradermal injection of PRP,
- Group B received chemical reconstruction of skin scars,
- and Group C was treated by combined skin needling and PRP. Each patient underwent 3 sessions at 2-week intervals.

The 3 groups showed statistically highly significant improvement in the degree of acne scars after treatment No major adverse effects were observed in the studied groups.

This is the first study to use intradermal injection of PRP alone for the treatment of atrophic acne scars. The 3 modalities showed a promising efficacy and safety in the treatment of atrophic acne scars.[255]

PRP Therapy Facial (aka the Vampire Facial®)

Platelet Rich Plasma (PRP) which contains growth factors is obtained by drawing your blood. Your blood is then spun in a high speed

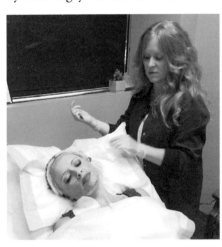

Michelle Darrow, RN, NP

centrifuge to separate the plasma from the red blood cells. Your face is then rolled with a derma roller. A derma roller is a cylindrical shaped drum that is studded with tiny fine "micro needles". Gently pricking your skin with the derma roller stimulates the creation of new skin cells and regeneration of damaged cells. Your own PRP is then massaged into the skin. The goal is to stimulate the production of collagen and elastin, and the creation of new cells. Your skin will glow and immediately feel smoother and softer, with progressive improvements continuing for several months.

Benefits include:

- Soften fine lines and wrinkles;
- Look refreshed and younger, with a more youthful skin texture, color and tone.

PRP Hair Growth

"PRP injection for androgenic alopecia is a simple, cost-effective and feasible treatment option for hair loss and can be regarded as a valuable adjuvant treatment modality for androgenic alopecia." [256]

Journal of Cutaneous and Aesthetic Surgery

Throughout this book we have documented the medical research and our own clinical experiences in utilizing Platelet Rich Plasma Therapy to regenerate damaged joints. In this section we will discuss the role of PRP for hair growth.

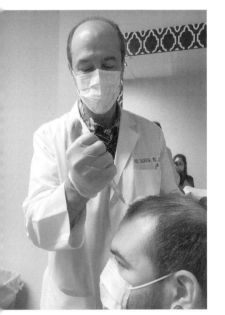

How PRP Stimulates Hair Growth

Platelet-rich plasma therapy stimulates hair growth through the promotion of vascularization and angiogenesis (the creation of new blood vessels that brings new blood circulation to the scalp), as well as encourages hair follicles to enter and extend the duration of the anagen phase (the most active growth portion of the hair growth cycle).[257]

Platelet rich plasma is concentrated blood plasma. In it is among the best weapons the immune system has to repair and regenerative tissue. These include platelet derived growth factor (PDGF), vascular endothelial growth factor (VEGF), transforming growth factor (TGF) and other bioactive proteins that aid in injury repair.

According to the National Institutes of Health:

Androgenetic alopecia is a common form of hair loss in both men and women. In men, this condition is also known as male-pattern baldness. Hair is lost in a well-defined pattern, beginning above both temples. Over time, the hairline recedes to form a characteristic "M" shape.

Hair also thins at the crown (near the top of the head), often progressing to partial or complete baldness.

The pattern of hair loss in women differs from male-pattern baldness. In women, the hair becomes thinner all over the head, and the hairline does not recede. Androgenetic alopecia in women rarely leads to total baldness.

In examining the benefits of PRP for hair growth, doctors at university medical centers in Greece published their review of PRP's effect on androgenetic alopecia and alopecia areata.

At the beginning of their paper, the Greek doctors answered a common question: why another hair loss treatment when there are so many to choose from?

Here is their answer: Despite available therapeutic options, the search for new, more effective hair restoration treatment is constant. Platelet-rich plasma could be the more effective treatment.

Growth factors in platelets' granules of PRP bind in the bulge area of hair follicle, promoting hair growth making PRP a potential useful therapeutic tool for alopecias, without major adverse effects.[258]

Doctors at the Santosh Medical College in India documented similar findings, in their study in the *Asian Journal of Transfusion Science*, the doctors conducted a study of 10 patients with hair loss. In the introduction of the study the doctors acknowledged that PRP has shown remarkable beneficial effects without any major adverse reactions in the treatment of androgenic alopecia, as did the Greek doctors.

Here is what the Indian doctors found:

The growth factors in autologous (your blood) PRP induces the proliferation of dermal papilla cells (Hair follicles). Ten patients were given PRP injections prepared from their own blood on the affected area of alopecia over a period of 3 months at intervals of 2–3 weeks and results were assessed. Three months after the treatment, the patients presented clinical improvement in the hair counts, hair thickness, hair root strength, and overall alopecia. They concluded that PRP appears to be a cheap, effective, and promising therapy for androgenic alopecia with no major adverse effects.[259]

In another study from Greek researchers, 20 patients, 18 males and 2 females, with androgenetic alopecia had three PRP treatment sessions performed every 21 days and a booster session at 6 months following the onset of therapy. At 6 months and at 1 year, hair volume was significantly increased.[260]

PRP vs. Minoxidil, Finasteride and Placebo

Doctors at university medical centers in Egypt compared topical minoxidil 5% and platelet rich plasma treatments for alopecia areata, a disease that results in one or more areas of coin-sized hairless patches.

Patients treated with minoxidil 5% and platelet rich plasma both had more significant hair growth than placebo.

Patients treated with platelet rich plasma had an earlier response in the form of hair regrowth, reduction in short vellus hair and dystrophic hair unlike patients treated with minoxidil and control.

With these findings the Egyptian doctors were able to conclude that platelet rich plasma is more effective in the treatment of alopecia areata than topical minoxidil 5%.[261]

In the citation at the beginning of this chapter from the *Journal of Cutaneous and Aesthetic Surgery,* Indian researchers at the SMT Kashibai Navale Medical College called PRP "a simple, cost-effective

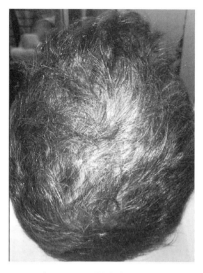

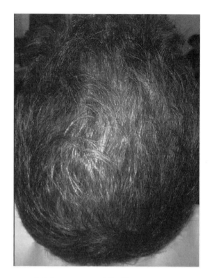

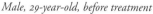

Male, 29-year-old, before treatment   *Male, 29-year-old, after treatment*

and feasible treatment option for hair loss." Here is what they based their opinion on:

> The doctors looked at patients suffering from androgenic alopecia and on topical *minoxidil* and *finasteride* for at least 6 months without much improvement. These patients were considered for PRP therapy which consisted of four treatments.
>
> After the 4th PRP treatment, a significant reduction in hair loss was observed between first and fourth injection as noticed by patients.

The study concludes: Treatment options for androgenic alopecia are very limited and include topical minoxidil and oral finasteride (FDA approved) either alone or in combination. However, there are several reported side effects such as headache and increase in other body hairs for minoxidil whereas loss of libido has been reported with oral finasteride. PRP injection for androgenic alopecia is a simple, cost-effective and feasible treatment option for hair.[263]

Doctors at the University of Rome reported their results of a randomized, placebo-controlled, half-head group study to compare the hair regrowth with PRP versus placebo.

In this study of three treatment cycles, the patients presented clinical improvement in the mean number of hairs, with a mean increase of 33.6 hairs in the target area and a mean increase in total hair density of 45.9 hairs per square centimeter compared with baseline values.

No side effects were noted during treatment. The data clearly highlight the positive effects of PRP injections on male pattern hair loss and absence of major side effects.[264]

Do you have questions about PRP and hair growth?
Call our office: 800-300-9000

Stories from our Patients

Betsy Cantor

My passion for long distance running began in the 1980's. After watching the 1984 Women's Olympic Marathon in Los Angeles I was inspired to attempt one myself. The running boom had just begun for women, and most people thought I was nuts. Fortunately, I was born with the essential traits of a marathon runner—stubbornness, perseverance, a sense of humor, humility, patience, and a pioneer spirit. Since those early days, I have completed over 25 marathons, 13.1 races, 10k's, you name it. I ran 6–7 days a week for years and when I trained for a marathon my monthly miles totaled at about 200.

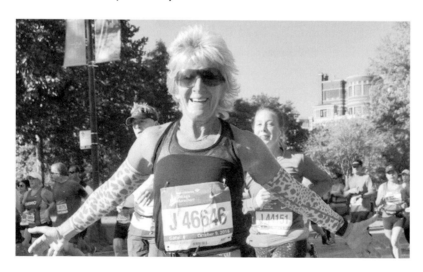

Several days after the 2014 LA Marathon I experienced severe pain and chronic swelling in the right knee after a "recovery" run. This began a never-ending series of orthopedic visits, physical therapy consultations, sports medicine opinions, acupuncture and even a miserable conversation with a noted sports radio doctor. An MRI and exam revealed lateral and medial meniscus tears, a bakers' cyst, arthritis and patella tracking issues. The opinions varied—arthroscopic surgery, pain medication and injections, an eventual knee replacement, and other bad news. Every professional told me the same thing about running "your running days are over—find something else to do". If you are a runner yourself, or a very active person you understand how it feels to constantly hear a prognosis of doom. My condition was explained as age related degeneration with no hope of returning to a high activity level. Labeling me as "degenerative" was more than I could take and the idea of never running again was not acceptable. Marathon runners are hard headed, so after about a year of this nonsense I stopped listening and started researching.

The PRP treatment option came to my attention as I learned more about alternatives available to professional athletes. It seemed futuristic and unattainable, and then one day I heard Dr. Darrow on the radio. He discussed his procedures with the radio audience and described using PRP and stem cell therapy as an alternative to surgery. Per Dr. Darrow, PRP was a process for rejuvenation and I loved the idea of healing without operating.

I set up a consultation with Dr. Darrow and his team. The first visit was an in-depth evaluation. Dr. Darrow spent a significant amount of time discussing my knee, running, treatment options and much more. I was impressed not only with his caring demeanor but also his upbeat attitude. He spoke about enabling a rejuvenation of the injured area by injecting my own perfect platelets into the knee. The process was explained in depth and it made total sense. Negative words such as deterioration or degeneration never entered the conversation, so for the first time in a long time I was optimistic.

PRP treatments began for me in 2015. After one treatment, I felt better and returned a couple of months later for two more. Dr. Darrow uses an ultra sound to find the exact location for the shot and is a masterful physician. The process is painless. As the platelets were injected I felt an overwhelming jolt of energy into my knee joint which I cannot explain logically. It just happened.

The recovery instructions are easy. You must rest the area completely and allow yourself enough time to heal. Dr. Darrow does not give exercises, and cautions against a hasty return to activity. He believes maintaining a healthy weight is key because it reduces the amount of stress on the joints. When I asked about running he made no promises and recommended I make upcoming fitness plans wisely. He encouraged me to reflect on the circumstances in my life which led to the injury, and remember PRP is not a protection against future over training.

As time went on the pain, swelling and stiffness disappeared and I began low impact cardio. I am a trainer and a Pilates teacher so I put myself on a strength program which would support my return to running. My initial goal was a few painless miles and eventually I got my wish. Racing and long distances were not on my radar, but soon I discovered how my patience and determination would lead to accomplishments beyond my own expectations.

Fast forward to the present. At 62 I feel rejuvenated and in the best shape of my life. I recently completed my 26th big city marathon in Chicago which was a miracle. Ten months after the last injection I ran the NYC half marathon and a month before I completed the LA Marathon 13.1 mile relay. Getting back to this level of physical activity came with hard work, grueling training and dedication on my part. I can take pride in my persistence and resolve. However, the act of healing and confidence in my ability to recover began with Dr. Darrow and his wonderful team. I am grateful every day to Dr. Darrow not only for the brilliant medical care, but also for his exceptional insight and guidance throughout the treatment process. Today I experience every run as a blessing, and I cannot wait to see what tomorrow has in store.

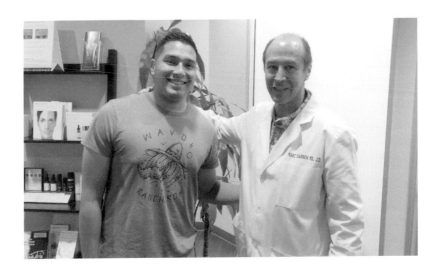

Andy Sanchez

I started seeing Dr. Darrow in late September for a nagging hip injury I had sustained while running and making an awkward step. This awkward step led to the muscles around my hip tightening. The muscle in front of my hip was constantly tight and my hip would make a snapping and cracking noise whenever I would flex my knee or rotate my leg. This pain made it unbearable to run. I was a bit skeptical at injections of PRP being able to help me out but I thought I'd give it a try since cortisone injections and physical therapy gave me little to no relief of my pain and stiffness.

I began feeling some relief about 11 days of my first PRP injection which was a great sign! I had my second treatment 14 days after my first one and it did take a bit longer to kick in but slowly but surely the healing process started! I currently feel 80% healed and had my third and hopefully last treatment of PRP today! I feel great and am sure that I will be back running soon!

Prolotherapy takes a while and you must be patient though. Follow Doc's orders to the tee in order to maximize your rate of healing. I found that keeping a healthy diet, getting adequate sleep, and taking the suggested supplements really aided my healing process. I hope this helps anyone who is thinking about starting a Prolotherapy treatment plan!

Dr. Darrow is the best and is very accessible! He gives patients his cell phone and urges patients to contact him if they have any questions about their healing process. This is awesome and he really does make an effort to answer all questions and guide you through the healing process! To top it off his staff is extremely professional and polite!

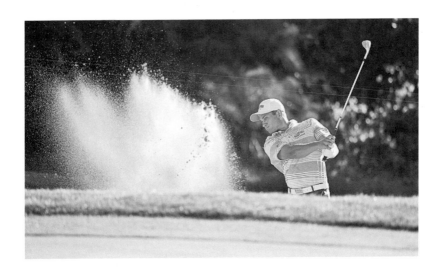

Alex Romo

When Alex Romo developed a problem in his neck, doctors told him that his golf career was over. Using an alternative stem cell therapy, the Oxnard resident is ready to resume his dream of playing on the PGA Tour.

THE VENTURA COUNTY STAR

December 8, 2015

Alex Romo thought he had it all figured out.

After graduating from Cal Poly San Luis Obispo in 2014, Romo spent that summer playing in his final amateur events in preparation of turning professional in the fall.

A week before his inaugural professional event, Romo woke up with significant pain in the left side of his neck and shoulder area. The Oxnard resident figured he had just slept wrong. As the days wore on, the pain persisted.

Despite the pain, Romo teed it up at the Bunker's Back Nine tournament at Camarillo Springs, but he didn't last long. His first full swing caused him so much pain he was forced to stop.

It turned out to be the last full swing the Villanova Prep graduate would take for 14 months due to an uncommon injury to his sterno-clavicular joint, a little-known joint between the sternum and clavicle. While he went through a long period where it looked like he might never fully recover, Romo stayed positive and kept looking for answers.

Two weeks ago he played his first pain-free round since the summer of 2014 and he's optimistic of playing on the PGA Tour someday.

"It's been a long road to get to this point, but I feel good and I'm excited about getting a second chance to pursue my dreams in golf," Romo said.

The process started with tests and consultations with various orthopedic doctors. It was determined the ligaments and tendons on the joint that connects the sternum and shoulder were stretched and frayed.

The cause of the injury was never fully determined, but doctors told Romo it was more than likely caused by overuse of the shoulder from things like weight lifting and swinging a golf club 100 mph.

"At some point the joint wore out and became unstable," Romo said. "Any time I would rotate and open my chest, I would hear a popping and clicking sound that was followed by crippling pain. In addition to the joint, I had a disc in the shoulder that also tore."

Surgery to replace the old tendons and ligaments with new ones taken from a cadaver was one way to solve the problem. But because the area where the joint is located is surrounded by critical arteries, including the carotid artery, doctors believed the surgery was too risky.

Doctors advised him to keep from using the joint as much as possible, with the hope that the rest would reduce the pain, but also said a return to golf was unlikely.

With the support of his parents Rick and Marianne, Romo started searching for alternative healing methods. Romo came across Dr. Marc Darrow, a doctor in West Los Angeles who uses stem cell therapy and platelet rich plasma therapy (PRP) to regenerate ligaments and tendons.

Darrow told Romo he had never seen an injury like the one Romo had, so he wasn't sure if his treatment would fully work. There was also the issue that both procedures are deemed experimental, so neither was covered by insurance.

"I had spent six months looking for other options, but the stem cell and PRP therapy seemed like the best option, even with the cost," Romo said. "I started with the stem cell, so they took bone marrow from my lower back and then reinjected the cells into my collarbone.

"It was really painful and left my back so sore it was hard to sit or even lay down. So I moved on the PRP therapy. We did 12 sessions from March through July."

After the last session, Romo stayed away from most physical activity to give the joint time to heal.

In the last month, he started lightly chipping balls and putting. The pain was gone, and over the last weeks Romo has slowly ramped up his activity. Two weeks ago he hit his first bucket of balls, and days later played his first round in 14 months.

"Those first few swings I was a little apprehensive, but so far it's been OK," Romo said. "I'm keeping things slow, but I've got my schedule in place for 2016 and to start chasing my dream again. I still have a ways to go, but I am excited about getting to this point. It hasn't been easy, but I'm optimistic about things moving forward."

Moving forward—a follow up

I took my son Alex Romo to see Dr. Marc Darrow back in February 2015 at one of the lowest points in his entire life and the work he's done for him has turned everything around. He had just finished his college golf career at Cal Poly SLO and was getting ready to turn professional in September of 2014. A week before his first tournament, he woke up with a weird pain near his left collarbone which has sidelined him from golf for the past 14 months. We would eventually learn that the joint connecting his left collarbone and sternum (sternoclavicular joint) was unstable and the tendons and ligaments surrounding it were loose, making it impossible for him to swing a golf club without pain. We spent 6 months consulting with different doctors and tried every treatment we could find. Cortisone shots, physical therapy, deep tissue massage, chiropractic . . . nothing seemed to help. It was as though he had a career ending injury on his hands and he was beyond devastated to see his life-long dream of playing golf on the PGA tour go out the window.

Then Dr. Darrow came into the picture. He consulted with us for hours on our first visit and then we decided to begin a series of both stem cell and PRP treatments. We had been considering surgery and Prolotherapy and had consulted with a number of orthopedic specialists previously, but finally felt the connection we were looking for with Dr. Darrow that made us comfortable enough to begin the treatment. He listened exceptionally well and really took his time to understand exactly what Alex was going through. We really appreciated this personal touch because his injury was very uncommon and difficult to explain and in most doctors' offices we had felt rushed and misunderstood when trying to tell Alex's story. As busy as we know Dr. Darrow is, he never once conveyed a sense of hurry to us and was beyond gracious with his time during every single treatment session. It was a very big decision for our family to try this experimental treatment that was both very costly and not guaranteed to heal Alex, but Dr. Darrow played a huge role in helping us decide on the best method of treatment and never pushed us into anything. He simply guided us through the process and offered advice when we asked for it. There was also the issue of some major arteries being located very close to the joint he was receiving injections in, but Dr. Darrow's touch with a needle was incredibly precise and steady and we always felt like Alex was in good hands. He got the treatments over as quickly and painlessly as possible every time.

We know from experience now that Dr. Darrow is an exceptionally talented doctor, but an even better person. He treats his patients like family and truly cares about the work he does and understands the power it has to heal. He makes you feel like your dream is his dream when he's treating you and I don't think that is something that can be faked. Only someone who genuinely cares about helping his patients heal and pours his heart and soul into what he does could make you feel as cared for as he does. We both became great friends with him throughout the series of visits for treatment. Even though Alex's situation was very serious and the outcome of the treatments would dictate his future, Dr Darrow kept it light and always chatted about golf and the newest swing tips he had read about or heard. The entire experience from start to finish with Dr. Darrow and his staff was an absolute pleasure. Alex remembers going through his first round of stem cell injections and being a bit scared to have bone marrow drilled from his back, but an assistant rubbed his shoulders throughout the whole process to help comfort him which was a huge help. He has never received a higher level of care at a doctor's office in his life.

Most importantly, we believe the treatments really did work because Alex has just recently returned to playing golf! After he finished his series of treatments in July, he began slowly easing back into working out and hitting golf balls and he played his first full round of golf in 14 months the day before Thanksgiving with me. We have professional tournaments lined up beginning in January of 2016 and plan to return to golf at the highest level in spite of this setback and guess what; I will get my caddie job back! Dr. Darrow is trying to help set Alex up with coaches that can teach him to swing the golf club in a more stress free way. Alex and I look forward to playing a round of golf with Dr. Darrow soon. In actuality, we will never be able to repay him for the help he's given us. He gave Alex his life back, a second chance at pursuing his dream, and for that we will be forever indebted to him.

http://archive.vcstar.com/sports/golf/alternative-treatment-helps-romo-get-back-on-course-258b2b22-7101-16b4-e053-0100007f8894-361127011.html

George Chung

I had been having progressively worse knee
pains on both knees for the past 6 years, having been a skier, love skiing bumps and also
jumps in the park, was on skis almost every
month of the year either skiing or training on
bumps or jumps for 10+ years while in my 40s,
in addition to racquetball, basketball, spin,
cycling & weights. All the abuse finally caught
up to me. I am now in my 50s. Tried to keep
them going by working out in spin classes &
with heavier weights 2–3 times a week, but the
pain had just gotten worse. Finally July of last
year, my left knee gave out, I was walking like
a handicapped person for a few days, which
really scared me. Did MRIs on both knees
(2nd for left & 1st on right), confirmed I was
very close to bone on bone on both & was a
knee replacement candidate on left, right not

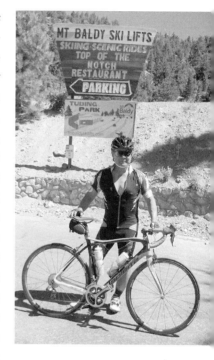

too far behind, with all sorts of issues, degenerative, bone contusions,
etc. Started research into better ways of cure than knee replacement
surgeries which I was trying to avoid at all cost.

After visiting the first Prolotherapy doctor in Santa Monica once
and not impressed by his office nor his much higher stem cell price,
I found Dr. Darrow. From the first visit, I just felt I have come to the
right place. Dr. Darrow puts you at ease right away, his staff is very
professional and friendly and all have been there a while. He examined my knees, saw the MRIs, knew exactly the course of the treatment. The wonderful staff explained to me fully the costs,etc. which
is all on his website anyway.No hidden cost. no surprises. No, the
insurance doesn't cover the treatment,but I did not want any surgery.
Looking back, this was by far the best option for me, with the BEST
DOCTOR!! Having researched (thank you google), read a lot into all
the articles I can get my hands on, and believing in the science behind
it, I decided to follow his instructions 100%. First two months, with

several stem cell & PRP injections, I did not try to push my legs at all. In fact, I just rested them most of the time, which is exactly what was recommended. Being an active person, that really bothered me at first. I also stopped taking Ibuprofen, which I used to take religiously. I have not taken them since, don't need them anymore! Also learned it prohibits healing. I traveled to Asia on an 11 day tour with lots of hikes 5 months into the treatment, a bit much now thinking back. I actually got back to skiing 6 months later, although only on groomed & 1 moderate run in the moguls each day, and resumed cycling & spin. 7 months into the treatments. Now, 17 months, multiple stem cells and PRP sessions later (just had a PRP yesterday—3 months after the last stem cell session, and I have been pushing the knees hard the last three months), I am working out 2–3 times a week in the gym, spin and weights. Just completed my first century (100 mile) ride from Orange County to San Diego two weeks ago. Also climbed on my road bikes up GMR, Chrystal Lake, Mt. Wilson, and Mt. Baldy many times (25–38 miles of climbing rides), and I rode three out of six days this week, 38 miles climbing, 82 miles flat, and 55 miles flat. Skied Mammoth three weeks ago on their opening weekend, my normal pace on groomed, fast GS, short radius turns, etc. The best thing is, now, I do all this without pain!! All the old pains, walking down stairs, sleeping (had to have a pillow under my knees), etc., or just walking in general, they are history!! Gone!! As I said, I do full workouts (but no more basketball) in the gym to support my active lifestyle just like before, which is very important if you are active to make sure your muscles are strong to support the repaired and regenerated knees.

Dr. Darrow has my highest recommendation!! I talked about my stem cell procedures and Dr. Darrow to all my friends and riding buddies. Although I have found that many people, even physicians (including several doc friends) do not have much knowledge of this procedure, including my roommate at the Asia trip, who is a kidney specialist, thus they termed it "experimental," "unproven," etc. All I can say is for me, and two of my dear friends who are 79 and 70 years old (shoulder and knee problems), without question, stem cell and PRP worked for us!! Thank you very much Dr. Darrow and all the staff for giving me a new lease (knees) on life. :)

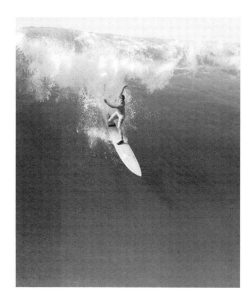

Nic Lamb, World Surfing Legend

(at the time of this writing ranked number 5 in the world)

"The stem and prp treatment I received from Dr. Darrow was truly incredible in how quickly I healed and returned back to my sport."

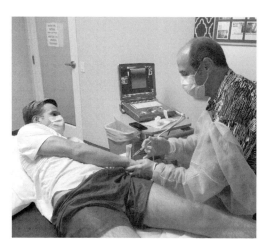

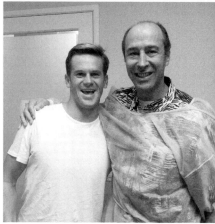

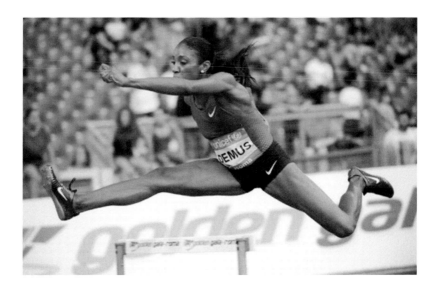

Lashinda Demus

- Olympic hurdler in the 400 meters
- 2011 world champion and 2012 Olympic silver medalist
- 2002 NCAA Outdoor champion
- 2003 NCAA Indoor 400m champion
- 2006 Outdoor Visa champion
- 2009 World Outdoor 4x400m gold medalist
- 2011 World Outdoor gold medalist
- Four-time USA Outdoor 400mH champion

Treated after 2012 Olympics for plantar fasciitis, knee ligaments and meniscus.

Jon Fro

After successful stem cells on my left knee in February, I returned to Dr. Darrow on March 21, 2016 to have stem cells in my back. Everything went great and all pain gone from my back so far. I have spinal stenosis.

My back is slightly stiff due to inactivity, however soon will be stretching and riding my bicycle :)

Dr. Darrow and his staff and wonderful folks . . . Whether you live in sunny California or over in Texas . . . the trip is worth it. I plan to return this summer if necessary for another treatment :)

By the way, my wife had stem in her left knee also plus vampire facelift and stem in her face. OMG . . . she loves Michelle Darrow also!!

John
Plano, Texas

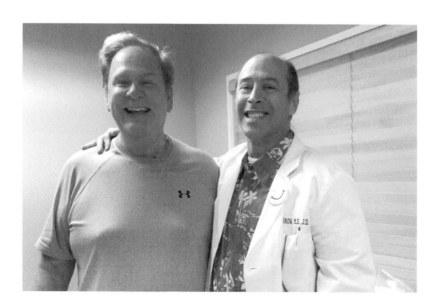

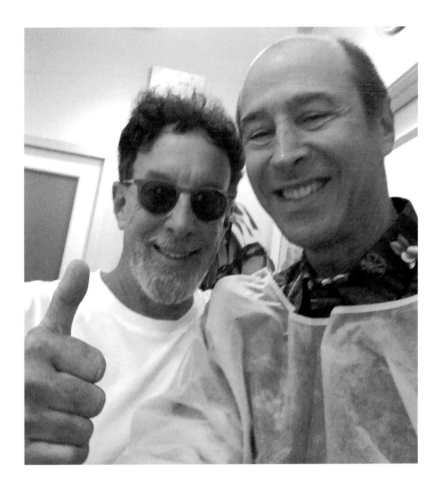

Mark Canton

Produced *300* and *300: Rise of an Empire.*

He was ready for shoulder surgery and saved by stem cells and PRP treatment.

Pauline Nordin

Dr. Darrow is leading the industry with his treatments and practice. As the founder of Fighter Diet I've made my body my paycheck, inspiring and motivating millions of fitness minded individuals around the world, and that's why getting help to speed up recovery when injuries strike are extremely helpful. I've trained for more than 18 years non-stop and I intend on continuing that all my life. The new technology of PRP and stem cells will assist me in this pursuit. We only have one body and it's critical to treat it like a racing car. Now and then it will break down since pushing to max is part of the deal to achieve excellence, and that's when I call Dr. Darrow, both to prevent further damage and to rejuvenate my body with its own inborn ability and talent.

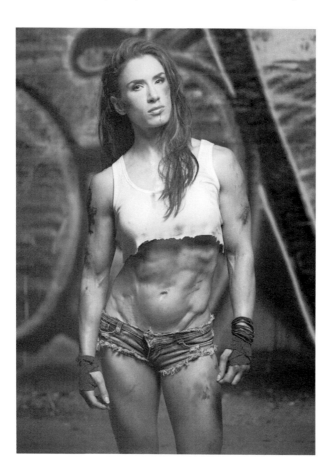

Yelp Reviews

Dan B. | Yelp

If only every doctor was like Dr. Darrow. I can't think of any other doctor who is willing to invest so much time talking to patients and answering their questions. Dr. Darrow truly has a passion for helping his patients heal. If you are in pain, I strongly suggest you at least investigate PRP and/or Stem Cell injections. If you look into these procedures, you would be doing yourself a disservice if you don't at least talk to Dr. Darrow. I don't think you will find another doctor with as much experience in this field as Dr. Darrow.

My son is a high school pitcher who went to Dr. Darrow after months of pain in his throwing arm. Over the summer he was diagnosed with a small tear in his UCL. Fortunately it was not big enough to even consider Tommy John surgery. The orthopedist we were seeing suggested months of rest and physical therapy and if that did not work we could try PRP. After a long layoff, the arm improved, but not 100% as there was still pain when throwing from certain arm slots. My son did not want to have another long layoff and roll the dice that this time would be different and time and physical therapy would do the trick. He wanted to do something proactive, so we started to seriously investigate PRP. This Orthopedist practice we were seeing although very well respected, was new to PRP and only had one doctor in their practice starting to use PRP. This was a concern, since I did not want my son to be part of this doctors learning curve.

This is when I found Dr. Darrow. We emailed him and he actually responded—I don't know of any doctors who respond to emails and do it quickly. After several emails back and forth answering many of my questions, we decided to have an office consultation. During the initial office visit, we decided to have the procedure done. However, the procedure we decided on was not PRP. Instead, we opted for Stem Cell injections. I was amazed that my son was able to get the injections on this visit. Base on my experience with other doctors, I was expecting to make another appointment weeks if not months out in the future. My son was so glad to have the injections done right away and not delay the road to recovery.

I am now glad to report that he is back to pitching pain free with better velocity than ever! Now I know why so many MLB pitchers are opting for PRP or Stem Cells rather than go under the Tommy John knife. This is the new frontier for medicine and we are so fortunate to have a pioneer in this field in Southern California.

Shawn H. | Yelp

I took my mother in for a consultation for Stem Cell injection into her knee, we had seen other Doctors and after meeting Dr. Darrow we made the decision to go with him. His explanation of the process was very clear and his friendly personality made the decision easy. He also explained that it's not that complicated, other doctors made it seem like this was rocket science and then put a hefty price tag on it to match. Dr. Darrow explained that he does this all day long and it takes 20 minutes tops of actual process. It was also offered at a reasonable price which allows one to have multiple treatments at his institute. I actually watched the entire process, the removal of the stem cells from hip bone and injection 20 minutes later of the concentrated stem cells and platelets into my mom's knee. She walked out of the doctors office a couple of hours later with the treatment we were looking for at a great price. It was a success as far as I can tell. Plus, they make you feel really comfortable in this office, nice people, they are not trying to trick anybody. They are just trying to treat their patients with the best treatments and service at a reasonable price, and most important they do it with a smile!! Thank you Dr. Darrow and staff.

Phillip Mac O. | Yelp

In April of 2015, I accidentally met Dr. Marc Darrow of the Darrow Stem Cell Institute at a golf course in West Los Angeles. I'm not one to believe in fate or destiny, but the lucky stars were in my pocket on that day and every day since. I'm a former professional athlete (PGA Tour Player). My age is sixty-four. I've never taken my health for granted. And I've always exercised diligently throughout my lifetime. Eighteen years ago, I had surgery on both of my knees to repair meniscus tears. The surgery was a resounding success. But for the last two and half years, my knees have slowly deteriorated (perhaps it's the aging process). They always feel swollen. I've lost range of motion, and they ache, even when I sleep. Worst yet, I couldn't exercise my legs even minimally anymore. My legs went from being the strongest part of my body, to the weakest anatomical link. You can imagine how destructive it was for me to play tournament golf. I couldn't. I had to stop playing. I had an MRI image study performed about a year ago and the radiology report was not favourable. I contacted a Doctor of Orthopaedic's in Buffalo, N.Y. (professional hockey team doctor) who performed surgery on me in the past. I tried to organise a surgical date, but his schedule was full for the next two weeks and he was leaving on a one week vacation thereafter. So I had to wait until his return. It was during this time, I met Dr. Darrow. He suggested that stem cell regenerative medicine may be an option to look into. On a professional level, I have personally funded and researched a scientific project on the biomechanics of the golf swing for over thirty years. So in my social education on medical science, I'm quite familiar with stem cell therapy and its possible benefits. So when I met Dr. Darrow, he didn't have to do much to convince me regenerative sports medicine might be viable option to pursue. On the flip side, Dr. Darrow informed me the injections may not work. He carefully explained this fact to me. But, despite this realization, I decided to have the stem cell injections performed. Ten months have passed since I had the first of three separate injections that were spaced out over a two month period between each successive injection. The results have been remarkable and extraordinary for me. Within a few days of the first injection, the swelling in my knees began to subside. I noticed I could walk up & down stairs with better mobility. Also, it was the first time in years, I slept painless throughout the night without having to wake up to the throbbing in my knees. The chronic pain was gone and I could feel I had greater range of motion. Yes, I could begin to squat again without having difficulty in getting up. The transformation was real and so unexpected in such a short time. Dr. Darrow asked me to follow a strict regimen of allowing plenty of time for the knees to rest before doing any exercise. I waited for thirty days before I put any kind of physical restraints on the connective tissue or muscles except for walking. When I started up on the exercise routine, I began by riding a stationary bicycle for ten minutes each day for a week. Then, I jogged slowly for ten minutes. I had no complications whatsoever either on the bicycle or after the run. I followed the same exercise protocols after each injection. This may be a reason why I've had such good short or long term results.

In closing, I can only speak for myself, regenerative sports medicine (stem cell injections) worked for me. I would recommend it for anyone to look into it before you had any surgery performed. I'm not saying, surgery is bad. But you may have a better result without having to be cut into and to compromise the surrounding anatomy in ways you can't see, but you can feel. I've had twelve surgeries on my body over the last twenty years. I question now, how much better off I may have been, if I had known the true benefits of regenerative medicine and stem cell therapy. Now, ten months later, after three injections, I can walk eighteen holes again, run again, and feel good again. I feel my chronological age has been pushed back a minimum of twenty years. How do I say thank you to Dr. Darrow and his conscientious staff for helping and assisting me with their knowledge, compassion and empathy in every little baby step I took along the way. I'm ready to start playing in tournaments again. All because of the conscientious pre-eminent research performed by scientists all over the world who truly understand regenerative medicine and that it is the wave of the future that is already here today in our modern society of the 21st century.

Best Regards,
Phillip Mac O

Stay T. | Yelp

Dr. Darrow treated my mother's knees with stem cell treatments these past two months. This was not an easy decision. We were looking at two other surgical options. We did not like any of them.

She has Osteoarthritis, and both knees are basically shot. The cartilage cushion is non-existing according to other doctors. Her walk confirms it is true, and it is difficult to observe.

Back at the hospital where she works, they recommended knee surgery for both knees. This meant cutting into the knee cap and connecting bone and capping them in with metal. This translated to being bed-ridden for about 6 months per knee. Not to mention the misery and pain involved. It was a daunting thought.

My mother is a very active person. She works at a hospital where she moves plenty and sees plenty. Only this time she would be the patient.

She just couldn't see herself falling apart like that. The thought was unbearable, and frankly depressing. She needed an alternative solution to keep going, and to keep moving. She needed Stem Cell to regenerate tissue.

This was not going to be easy. She was going to have to travel from Arizona and ask for time off away from work to do so. Also, Stem Cell is not recognized by insurance companies. She needed the best doctor to do it, and one she could trust.

A family member recommended Dr. Darrow and his practice. Our family is extremely grateful she went to the Darrow Stem Cell Institute. The staff is one amazing team. They are helpful, and will answer questions to your satisfaction. They each take extra care to make sure you are comfortable and a priority. They know that such a procedure can be intrusive and painful. They do an amazing job of working swiftly and accurately to make sure the procedure is a success. They cover the bases to make sure you understand how it works, what it involves and what recuperation means to the patient after the procedure. They explain the recovery steps and what you need to do and not do for your wellness. They provide you a list of what you can take orally for pain management and healthy living.

We were skeptical, but that went away. The first treatment was applied to her left knee. She will continue her treatments with Dr. Darrow for sure. Mom has gained an understanding, and a deep appreciation for Dr. Darrow's service and that of his staff. These are very caring people despite the jackets, gloves and masks. They each have a duty and frankly carry their heart on their sleeves. Be happy to meet such a wonderful team of persons to work with. This is a wonderful place with lots to offer including Stem Cell. They will take good care of you.

They are busy so make sure to plan ahead. There is a morning and afternoon appointment window time for Stem Cell application. Get ready for a very profound experience and getting your life back every step of the way.

It's obvious that not all patients heal from Regenerative Medicine (Stem Cells, PRP, Prolotherapy), surgery, or any type of medicine. If you look at all my Yelp.com reviews, you will also see complaints and my answers to them. Regenerative Medicine is not a panacea for healing, but in my mind, when applicable, the correct choice over drugs and surgery.

Notes

1. Nazempour A, Van Wie BJ. Chondrocytes, mesenchymal stem cells, and their combination in articular cartilage regenerative medicine. *Ann Biomed Eng.* 2016 May;44(5):1325-54. doi: 10.1007/s10439-016-1575-9. Epub 2016 Mar 17. Review.

2. Thorlund JB, C. B. Juhl CB, Roos EM, Lohmander LS. Arthroscopic surgery for degenerative knee: systematic review and meta-analysis of benefits and harms. *BMJ.* 2015; 2015 (Jun 16);350:h2747. doi: 10.1136/bmj.h2747.

3. Lenza M, Ferraz Sde B, Viola DC, Garcia Filho RJ, Cendoroglo Neto M, Ferretti M. Epidemiology of total hip and knee replacement: a cross-sectional study. *Einstein* (São Paulo). 2013 Apr-Jun;11(2):197-202.

4. Davatchi F, Sadeghi Abdollahi B, Mohyeddin M, Nikbin B. Mesenchymal stem cell therapy for knee osteoarthritis: 5 years follow-up of three patients. *Int. J. Rheum Dis.* 2015 May 20. doi: 10.1111/1756-185X.12670.

5. Zhang Q, Chen Y, Wang Q, Fang C, Sun Y, Yuan T, Wang Y, Bao R, Zhao N. Effect of bone marrow-derived stem cells on chondrocytes from patients with osteoarthritis. *Mol Med Rep.* 2016 Feb;13(2):1795-800. doi: 10.3892/mmr.2015.4720.

6. Huang S, Xu L, Zhang Y, Sun Y, Li G. Systemic and local administration of allogeneic bone marrow derived mesenchymal stem cells promotes fracture healing in rats. *Cell Transplant.* 2015; 24(12):2643-55. doi: 10.3727/096368915X687219.

7. Dhillon RS, Schwarz EM, Maloney MD. Platelet-rich plasma therapy—future or trend? *Arthritis Res Ther.* 2012 Aug 8;14(4):219. doi: 10.1186/ar3914.

8. Watson L et al. Local administration of non-diabetic MSCs to diabetic femoral fractures enhances callus remodelling and deposition of reparative bone. *End Abstr.* 2015; 37.

9. Titorencu I, Pruna V, Jinga VV, Simionescu M. Osteoblast ontogeny and implications for bone pathology: an overview. *Cell Tissue Res.* 2014 Jan;355(1):23-33. doi: 10.1007/s00441-013-1750-3. Epub 2013 Nov 29.

10. Calori GM, Mazza E, Colombo M, Mazzola S, Mineo GV, Giannoudis

PV. Treatment of AVN using the induction chamber technique and a bio-logical-based approach: Indications and clinical results. *Injury.* 2013 Sep 19. pii: S0020-1383(13)00423-3. doi: 10.1016/j.injury.2013.09.014. [Epub ahead of print.]

11. Hernigou P, Flouzat-Lachaniette CH, Delambre J, Poignard A, Allain J, Chevallier N, Rouard H. Osteonecrosis repair with bone marrow cell therapies: state of the clinical art. *Bone.* 2015 Jan;70:102-9. doi: 10.1016/j.bone.2014.04.034. Epub 2014 Jul 10.

12. Lau RL, Perruccio AV, Evans HM, Mahomed SR, Mahomed NN, Gandhi R. Stem cell therapy for the treatment of early stage avascular necrosis of the femoral head: a systematic review. *BMC Musculoskelet Disord.* 2014 May 16;15:156. doi: 10.1186/1471-2474-15-156. PubMed Abstract.

13. Qi Y, Feng G, Yan W. Mesenchymal stem cell-based treatment for cartilage defects in osteoarthritis. Mol Biol Rep. 2012 May;39(5):5683-9. Epub 2011 Dec 20.

14. Jakobsen RB, Shahdadfar A, Reinholt FP, Brinchmann JE. Chondrogenesis in a hyaluronic acid scaffold: comparison between chondrocytes and MSC from bone marrow and adipose tissue. *Knee Surg Sports Traumatol Arthrosc.* 2010 Oct;18(10):1407-16. doi: 10.1007/s00167-009-1017-4. Epub 2009 Dec 18. 2010 Oct;18(10):1407-16. doi: 10.1007/s00167-009-1017-4. Epub 2009 Dec 18. Erratum in: *Knee Surg Sports Traumatol Arthrosc.* 2014 Jul;22(7):1711-4.

15. Shafiee A, Seyedjafari E, Soleimani M, Ahmadbeigi N, Dinarvand P, Ghaemi N. A comparison between osteogenic differentiation of human unrestricted somatic stem cells and mesenchymal stem cells from bone marrow and adipose tissue. *Biotechnol Lett.* 2011 Jun;33(6):1257-64. doi: 10.1007/s10529-011-0541-8. Epub 2011 Feb 2.PubMed PMID: 21287233.

16. Frisbie DD, Kisiday JD, Kawcak CE, Werpy NM, McIlwraith CW. Evaluation of adipose-derived stromal vascular fraction or bone marrow-derived mesenchymal stem cells for treatment of osteoarthritis. *J Orthop Res.* 2009 Dec;27(12):1675-80. doi: 10.1002/jor.20933. PubMed PMID: 19544397.

17. Li Q, Tang J, Wang R, Bei C, Xin L, Zeng Y, Tang X. Comparing the chondrogenic potential in vivo of autogeneic mesenchymal stem cells derived from different tissues. *Artif Cells Blood Substit Immobil Biotechnol.* 2011 Feb;39(1):31-8. doi: 10.3109/10731191003776769. Epub 2010 Nov 30. PubMed PMID: 21117872.

18. Niemeyer P, Fechner K, Milz S, Richter W, Suedkamp NP, Mehlhorn AT, Pearce S, Kasten P. Comparison of mesenchymal stem cells from bone marrow and adipose tissue for bone regeneration in a critical size defect of the sheep tibia and the influence of platelet-rich plasma. *Biomaterials.* 2010 May;31(13):3572-9.

19. Vidal MA, Robinson SO, Lopez MJ, Paulsen DB, Borkhsenious O, Johnson JR, Moore RM, Gimble JM. Comparison of chondrogenic potential in equine mesenchymal stromal cells derived from adipose tissue and bone marrow. *Vet Surg.* 2008 Dec;37(8):713-24. doi: 10.1111/j.1532-950X.2008.00462.x. PubMed PMID: 19121166;PubMed Central PMCID: PMC2746327.

20. Chang YH, Liu HW, Wu KC, Ding DC. Mesenchymal stem cells and their clinical applications in osteoarthritis. *Cell Transplant.* 2015 Dec 18. [Epub ahead of print.]

21. He M, Gan AW, Lim AY, Goh JC, Hui JH, Chong AK. Bone marrow derived mesenchymal stem cell augmentation of rabbit flexor tendon healing. *Hand Surg.* 2015 Oct;20(3):421-9. doi: 10.1142/S0218810415500343.

22. Tetta C, Consiglio AL, Bruno S, Tetta E, Gatti E, Dobreva M, Cremonesi F, Camussi G. Muscles: the role of microvesicles derived from mesenchymal stem cells in tissue regeneration; a dream for tendon repair? *Ligaments Tendons J.* 2012 Oct 16;2(3):212-21. Print 2012 Jul.

23. Shapiro E, Grande D, Drakos M. Biologics in Achilles tendon healing and repair: a review. *Curr Rev Musculoskelet Med.* 2015 Feb 6. PubMed.

24. Pasquale MK, Louder AM, Cheung RY, Reiners AT, Mardekian J, Sanchez RJ, Goli V. Healthcare utilization and costs of knee or hip replacements versus pain-relief injections. *Am Health Drug Benefits* 2015 Oct;8(7):384-94.

25. Smith TO, Purdy R, Lister S, Salter C, Fleetcroft R, Conaghan PG. Attitudes of people with osteoarthritis towards their conservative management: a systematic review and meta-ethnography. *Rheumatol Int.* 2013 Dec 5. [Epub ahead of print.]

26. Orozco L, Munar A, Soler R, Alberca M, Soler F, Huguet M, Sentís J, Sánchez A, García-Sancho J. Treatment of knee osteoarthritis with autologous mesenchymal stem cells: a pilot study. *Transplantation.* 2013 May 15. [Epub ahead of print.]

27. Barry F, Murphy M. Mesenchymal stem cells in joint disease and repair. *Nat Rev Rheumatol.* 2013 Oct;9(10):584-94. doi: 10.1038/nrrheum.2013.109. Epub 2013 Jul 23.

28. Diekman BO, Guilak F. Stem cell-based therapies for osteoarthritis: challenges and opportunities. *Curr Opin Rheumatol.* 2013;25(1):119-126.

29. Dhillon RS, Schwarz EM, Maloney MD. Platelet-rich plasma therapy—future or trend? *Arthritis Res Ther.* 2012 Aug 8;14(4):219. [Epub ahead of print.]

30. Rodriguez IA, Growney Kalaf EA, Bowlin GL, Sell SA. Platelet-rich plasma in bone regeneration: engineering the delivery for improved clinical efficacy. *BioMed Res Int.* 2014;2014:392398. doi:10.1155/2014/392398

31. Oryan A, Alidadi S, Moshiri A Platelet-rich plasma for bone healing and regeneration. Expert Opin Biol Ther. 2015 Dec 4:1-20. [Epub ahead of print.]

32. Mattiello A, Cacciapuoti C. Autologous platelet gel improves bone reconstruction of large defects in patients with bone giant cell tumors. In Vi vo. 2015 Sep-Oct;29(5):533-540.

33. Civinini R, Macera A, Nistri L, Redl B, Innocenti M. The use of autologous blood-derived growth factors in bone regeneration. Clin Cases Miner Bone Metab. 2011 Jan-Apr; 8(1):25-31.

34. Nagaveni NB, Praveen RB, Umashankar KV, Pranav B, Sreedevi R, Radhika NB. Efficacy of platelet-rich plasma (PRP) in bone regeneration after cyst enucleation in pediatric patients—a clinical study. J Clin Pediatr Dent. 2010 Fall;35(1):81-7.

35. Civinini R, Nistri L, Martini C, Redl B, Ristori G, Innocenti M. Growth factors in the treatment of early osteoarthritis. *Clin Cases Miner Bone Metab*. 2013 Jan;10(1):26-9. doi: 0.11138/ccmbm/2013.10.1.026. PubMed Abstract.

36. Dallari D, Stagni C, Rani N, Sabbioni G, Pelotti P, Torricelli P, Tschon M, Giavaresi G. Ultrasound-guided injection of platelet-rich plasma and hyaluronic acid, separately and in combination, for hip osteoarthritis: a randomized controlled study. *Am J Sports Med*. 2016 Jan 21. pii: 0363546515620383. [Epub ahead of print]

37. Rafols C, Monckeberg JE, Numair J, Botello J, Rosales J. Platelet-rich plasma augmentation of arthroscopic hip surgery for femoroacetabular impingement: a prospective study with 24-month follow-up. *Arthroscopy*. 2015 Oct;31(10):1886-92. doi: 10.1016/j.arthro.2015.03.025. Epub 2015 May

38. Gullung GB, Woodall JW, Tucci MA, James J, Black DA, McGuire RA. Platelet-rich plasma effects on degenerative disc disease: analysis of histology and imaging in an animal model. *Evid Based Spine Care J*. 2011 Nov;2(4):13-8. doi: 10.1055/s-0031-1274752.

39. Khalaf K, Nikkhoo M, Ya-Wen Kuo, Yu-Chun Hsu, Parnianpour M, Campbell-Kyureghyan N, Haghpanahi M, Jaw-Lin Wang. Recovering the mechanical properties of denatured intervertebral discs through Platelet-Rich Plasma therapy. *Conf Proc IEEE Eng Med Biol Soc*. 2015 Aug; 933-6. doi: 10.1109/EMBC.2015.7318516.

40. Li M, Zhang C, Ai Z, Yuan T, Feng Y, Jia W. Therapeutic effectiveness of intra-knee-articular injection of platelet-rich plasma on knee articular cartilage degeneration. *Zhongguo Xiu Fu Chong Jian Wai Ke Za Zhi*. 2011 Oct;25(10):1192-6.

41. Wang-Saegusa A, Cugat R, Ares O, et al. Infiltration of plasma rich in growth factors for osteoarthritis of the knee short-term effects on function and quality of life. *Arch Orthop Trauma Surg*. 2011 Mar;131(3):311-7. Epub 2010 Aug 17.

42. Kanchanatawan W et al. Short-term outcomes of platelet-rich plasma injection for treatment of osteoarthritis of the knee. *Knee Surg Sports Traumatol*. Arthrosc. 2015 Sep 19. [Epub ahead of print]

43. Pourcho AM, Smith J, Wisniewski SJ, Sellon JL. Intraarticular platelet-rich plasma injection in the treatment of knee osteoarthritis: review and recommendations. *Am J Phys Med Rehabil*. 2014 Nov;93(11 Suppl 3):S108-21. doi: 10.1097/PHM.0000000000000115.

44. Sampson S, Reed M, Silvers H, et al. Injection of platelet-rich plasma in patients with primary and secondary knee osteoarthritis: a pilot study. *Am J Phys Med Rehabil*. 2010 Dec;89(12):961-9.

45. Blanke F, Vavken P, Haenle M, von Wehren L, Pagenstert G, Majewski M. Percutaneous injections of platelet-rich plasma for treatment of intrasubstance meniscal lesions. *Muscles Ligaments Tendons J*. 2015 Oct 20;5(3):162-166.

46. Campbell KA, Saltzman BM, Mascarenhas R, Khair MM, Verma NN, Bach BR Jr, Cole BJ. A Systematic Review of Overlapping Meta-analyses. *Arthroscopy*. 2015 Nov;31(11):2213-21. doi: 10.1016/j.arthro.2015.03.041. Epub 2015 May 29.

47. Wu CC, Chen WH, Zao B, Lai PL, Lin TC, Lo HY, Shieh YH, Wu CH, Deng WP. Regenerative potentials of platelet-rich plasma enhanced by collagen in retrieving pro-inflammatory cytokine-inhibited chondrogenesis. *Biomaterials*. 2011 Sep;32(25):5847-54. Epub 2011 May 25.

48. van Buul GM et al. Platelet-rich plasma releasate inhibits inflammatory processes in osteoarthritic chondrocytes. *Am J Sports Med*. 2011 Nov;39(11):2362-70. Epub 2011 Aug 19.

49. Kon E, Buda R, Filardo G, Di Martino A, Timoncini A, Canacchi A, Fornasari PM, Giannini S, Marcacci M. Platelet-rich plasma: intra-articular knee injections produced favorable results on degenerative cartilage lesions. *Knee Surg Sports Traumatol Arthrosc*. 2010; 18(4):472-479.

50. Gosens T, Den Oudsten BL, Fievez E, van 't Spijker P, Fievez A. Pain and activity levels before and after platelet-rich plasma injection treatment of patellar tendinopathy: a prospective cohort study and the influence of previous treatments. *Int Orthop*. 2012 Apr 27.

51. Mei-Dan O, Carmont MR. The role of platelet-rich plasma in rotator cuff repair. *Sports Med Arthrosc*. 2011 Sep;19(3):244-50. doi: 10.1097/JSA.0b013e318227b2dc.

52. von Wehren L, Blanke F, Todorov A, Heisterbach P, Sailer J, Majewski M. The effect of subacromial injections of autologous conditioned plasma versus cortisone for the treatment of symptomatic partial rotator cuff tears. *Knee Surg Sports Traumatol.Arthrosc*. 2015 May 28. [Epub ahead of print]

53. Yang J, Sun Y, Xu P, Cheng B. Can patients get better clinical outcomes by using PRP in rotator cuff repair: a meta-analysis of randomized controlled trials. *J Sports Med Phys Fitness*. 2015 Oct 16.

54. http://www.aaos.org/CustomTemplates/AcadNewsArticle.aspx?id=8767&ssopc=1

55. Salamanna F, Veronesi F. New and emerging strategies in platelet-rich plasma application in musculoskeletal regenerative procedures: general overview on still open questions and outlook. BioMed Research International. Volume 2015 (2015), Article ID 846045, 24 pages

56. Murray DJ, Javed S, Jain N, Kemp S, Watts AC. Platelet-rich plasma injections in treating lateral epicondylosis: a review of the recent evidence. *J Hand Microsurg*. 2015 Dec;7(2):320-325. Epub 2015 Jul 8.

57. Guelfi M, Pantalone A, Vanni D, Abate M, et al. Long-term beneficial effects of platelet-rich plasma for non-insertional Achilles tendinopathy. *Foot Ankle Surg*. 2015 Sep;21(3):178-81. doi: 10.1016/j.fas.2014.11.005. Epub 2014 Dec 11. PubMed Abstract.

58. López-Gavito E, Gómez-Carlín LA, Parra-Téllez P, Vázquez-Escamilla J. Platelet-rich plasma for managing calcaneus tendon tendinopathy and plantar fasciitis. *Acta Ortop Mex*. 2011 Nov-Dec;25(6):380-5. PubMed PRP Abstract.

59. Gaweda K, Tarczynska M, Krzyzanowski W. Treatment of Achilles tendinopathy with platelet-rich plasma. *Int J Sports Med*. 2010 Aug;31(8):577-83. Epub 2010 Jun 9. PubMed Abstract.

60. Hegab AF et al. Platelet-Rich Plasma Injection as an Effective Treatment

for Temporomandibular Joint Osteoarthritis. *J Oral Maxillofac Surg.* 2015 Sep;73(9):1706-13. doi: 10.1016/j.joms.2015.03.045. Epub 2015 Mar 24.

61. Hancı M, Karamese M, Tosun Z, Aktan TM, Duman S, Savacı N. Intra-articular platelet-rich plasma injection for the treatment of temporomandibular disorders and a comparison with arthrocentesis. *J Craniomaxillofac Surg.* 2015 Jan;43(1):162-6. doi: 10.1016/j.jcms.2014.11.002. Epub 2014 Nov 15.

62. Pihut M, Szuta M, Ferendiuk E, Zeńczak-Więckiewicz D. Evaluation of pain regression in patients with temporomandibular dysfunction treated by intra-articular platelet-rich plasma injections: a preliminary report. *Biomed Res Int.* 2014;2014:132369. doi: 10.1155/2014/132369. Epub 2014 Aug 3.

63. Salamanna F et al. New and emerging strategies in platelet-rich plasma application in musculoskeletal regenerative procedures: general overview on still open questions and outlook. *BioMed Res Int.* 2015. Article ID 846045.

64. Heldring N, Mäger I, Wood MJ, Le Blanc K, Andaloussi SE. Therapeutic potential of multipotent mesenchymal stromal cells and their extracellular vesicles. *Hum Gene Ther.* 2015 Aug;26(8):506-17. doi: 10.1089/hum.2015.072. Epub 2015 Aug 3. Review.

65. Beswick AD, Wylde V, Gooberman-Hill R. Interventions for the prediction and management of chronic postsurgical pain after total knee replacement: systematic review of randomised controlled trials. *BMJ Open.* 2015 May 12;5(5):e007387. doi: 10.1136/bmjopen-2014-007387.

66. Stacey D, et al. Impact of patient decision aids on appropriate and timely access to hip or knee arthroplasty for osteoarthritis: A randomized controlled trial. Osteoarthritis Cartilage. 2015 Aug 4. pii: S1063-4584(15)01267-4. doi: 10.1016/j.joca.2015.07.024.

67. Jones DL, Bhanegaonkar AJ, Billings AA, et al. Differences between actual and expected leisure activities after total knee arthroplasty for osteoarthritis. *J Arthroplasty.* 2012;27:1289–1296. doi: 10.1016/j.arth.2011.10.030.

68. Park CN, White PB, Meftah M, Ranawat AS, Ranawat CS. Diagnostic Algorithm for Residual Pain After Total Knee Arthroplasty. 2016 Mar 1;39(2):e246-52. doi: 10.3928/01477447-20160119-06. Epub 2016 Jan 25.

69. http://www.wiley.com/WileyCDA/PressRelease/pressReleaseId-111028.html

70. Katz JN. Appropriateness of total knee replacement. *Arthritis Rheumatol.* 2014 Aug; 66(8): 1979–1981. doi: 10.1002/art.38688.

71. Graichen H, Strauch M, Katzhammer T, Zichner L, von Eisenhart-Rothe R. Ligament instability in total knee arthroplasty—causal analysis. *Orthopade.* 2007 Jul;36:652–656. 650. PubMed.

72. Al-Hadithy N, Rozati H, Sewell MD, Dodds AL, Brooks P, Chatoo M. Causes of a painful total knee arthroplasty. Are patients still receiving total knee arthroplasty for extrinsic pathologies? *Int Orthop.* Epub. 2012 Jan 11.

73. Hah JM, Sharifzadeh Y, Wang BM, Gillespie MJ, Goodman SB, Mackey SC, Carroll IR. Factors Associated with Opioid Use in a Cohort of Patients Presenting for Surgery. *Pain Res. Treat.* 2015; 829696. Published online 2015 Dec 31. doi: 10.1155/2015/829696.

74. Zywiel MG, Stroh DA, Lee SY, Bonutti PM, Mont MA. Chronic opioid use prior to total knee arthroplasty. *J Bone Joint Surg Am.* 2011 Nov 2;93(21):1988-93. doi: 10.2106/JBJS.J.01473.

75. Thomazeau J, Rouquette A, Martinez V, Rabuel C, Prince N, Laplanche JL, Nizard R, Bergmann JF, Perrot S, Lloret-Linares C. Acute pain factors predictive of post-operative pain and opioid requirement in multimodal analgesia following knee replacement. *Eur J Pain.* 2015 Oct 30. doi: 10.1002/ejp.808.

76. Moucha CS, Weiser MC, Levin EJ. Current strategies in anesthesia and analgesia for total knee arthroplasty. *J Am Acad Orthop Surg.* 2016 Feb;24(2):60-73. doi: 10.5435/JAAOS-D-14-00259.

77. das Nair R, Anderson P, Clarke S, Leighton P, Lincoln NB, Mhizha-Murira JR, Scammell BE, Walsh DA. Home-administered pre-surgical psychological intervention for knee osteoarthritis (HAPPiKNEES): study protocol for a randomised controlled trial. *Trials.* 2016 Jan 27;17(1):54. doi: 10.1186/s13063-016-1165-z. PubMed PMID: 26818407; PubMed Central PMCID: PMC4730777.

78. Bierke S, Häner M, Petersen W. Influence of somatization and depressive symptoms on the course of pain within the first year after uncomplicated total knee replacement: a prospective study. *Int Orthop.* 2016 Jan 28. [Epub ahead of print.] PubMed PMID: 26820743.

79. Bistolfi A, Bettoni E, Aprato A, Milani P, Berchialla P, Graziano E, Massazza G, Lee GC. The presence and influence of mild depressive symptoms on post-operative pain perception following primary total knee arthroplasty. *Knee Surg Sports Traumatol Arthrosc.* 2015 Sep 21. [Epub ahead of print.]

80. Urquhart DM, Phyomaung PP, Dubowitz J, Fernando S, Wluka AE, Raajmaakers P, Wang Y, Cicuttini FM. Are cognitive and behavioural factors associated with knee pain? A systematic review. *Semin Arthritis Rheum.* 2015 Feb;44(4):445-55.

81. Phyomaung PP, Dubowitz J, Cicuttini FM, et al. Are depression, anxiety and poor mental health risk factors for knee pain? A systematic review. *BMC Musculoskeletal Disorders.* 2014;15:10. doi:10.1186/1471-2474-15-10.

82. Bardgett M, Lally J, Malviya A, Deehan D. Return to work after knee replacement: a qualitative study of patient experiences. *BMJ Open.* 2016;6:e007912. doi:10.1136/bmjopen-2015-007912.

83. Anderson JA, Little D, Toth AP, Moorman CT 3rd, Tucker BS, Ciccotti MG, Guilak F. Stem cell therapies for knee cartilage repair: the current status of preclinical and clinical studies. *Am J Sports Med.* 2014 Sep;42(9):2253-61. doi: 10.1177/0363546513508744. Epub 2013 Nov 12.

84. Vangsness CT Jr et al. Adult human mesenchymal stem cells delivered via intra-articular injection to the knee following partial medial meniscectomy: a randomized, double-blind, controlled study. *J Bone Joint Surg Am.* 2014 Jan 15;96(2):90-8. doi: 10.2106/JBJS.M.00058.

85. Kanchanatawan W et al. Short-term outcomes of platelet-rich plasma injection for treatment of osteoarthritis of the knee. *Knee Surg Sports Traumatol Arthrosc.* 2015 Sep 19. [Epub ahead of print]

86. Hsu WK, Mishra A, Rodeo SR, Fu F, Terry MA, Randelli P, Canale ST, Kelly FB. Platelet-rich plasma in orthopaedic applications: evidence-based recommendations for treatment. *J Am Acad Orthop Surg*. 2013 Dec;21(12):739-48. doi: 10.5435/JAAOS-21-12-739.

87. Sun Y, Feng Y, Zhang CQ, Chen SB, Cheng XG. The regenerative effect of platelet-rich plasma on healing in large osteochondral defects. *Int Orthop*. 2010 Apr;34(4):589-97. Epub 2009 May 12.

88. Li M, Zhang C, Ai Z, Yuan T, Feng Y, Jia W. Therapeutic effectiveness of intra-knee-articular injection of platelet-rich plasma on knee articular cartilage degeneration. *Zhongguo Xiu Fu Chong Jian Wai Ke Za Zhi*. 2011 Oct;25(10):1192-6.

89. Richter DL, Schenck RC Jr, Wascher DC, Treme G. Knee articular cartilage repair and restoration techniques: a review of the literature. *Sports Health*. 2015 Oct 12. pii: 1941738115611350. [Epub ahead of print.]

90. Campbell AB, Pineda M, Harris JD, Flanigan DC. Return to sport after articular cartilage repair in athletes' knees: a systematic review. *Arthroscopy*. 2015 Oct 30. pii: S0749-8063(15)00706-9. doi: 10.1016/j.arthro.2015.08.028. [Epub ahead of print.]

91. Kane P, Frederick R, Tucker B. Surgica l restoration/repair of articular cartilage injuries in athletes. *Phys Sportsmed*. 2013 May;41(2):75-86. doi: 10.3810/psm.2013.05.2017.

92. K Srinivas Rao Proof of concept, engineered cartilage tissue for cartilage injuries of knee. *Saudi Journal of Sports Medicine* 2014:14:2:155-157

93. Sánchez M, Anitua E, Orive G, Mujika I, Andia I. Platelet-rich therapies in the treatment of orthopaedic sport injuries. *Sports Med*. 2009;39(5):345-54.doi: 10.2165/00007256-200939050-00002.

94. Ehrenfest DM, Bielecki T, Mishra A, Borzini P, Inchingolo F, Sammartino G, Rasmusson L, Evert PA. In search of a consensus terminology in the field of platelet concentrates for surgical use: platelet-rich plasma (PRP), platelet-rich fibrin (PRF), fibrin gel polymerization and leukocytes.

95. Pestka JM, Feucht MJ, Porichis S, Bode G, Südkamp NP, Niemeyer P. Return to sports activity and work after autologous chondrocyte implantation of the knee: which factors influence outcomes? *Am J Sports Med*. 2015 Dec 9. pii: 0363546515614578. [Epub ahead of print.]

96. Mobasheri A, Kalamegam G, Musumeci G, Batt ME. Chondrocyte and mesenchymal stem cell-based therapies for cartilage repair in osteoarthritis and related orthopaedic conditions. *Maturitas*. 2014 Jul;78(3):188-198. doi: 10.1016/j.maturitas.2014.04.017. Epub 2014 May 2. PubMed.

97. Tay LX, Ahmad RE, Dashtdar H, Tay KW, Masjuddin T, Ab-Rahim S, Chong PP, Selvaratnam L, Kamarul T. Treatment outcomes of alginate-embedded allogenic mesenchymal stem cells versus autologous chondrocytes for the repair of focal articular cartilage defects in a rabbit model. *Am J Sports Med*. 2012 Jan;40(1):83-90. Epub 2011 Sep 13. PubMed.

98. Zhang Q, Chen Y, Wang Q, Fang C, Sun Y, Yuan T, Wang Y, Bao R, Zhao N. Effect of bone marrow-derived stem cells on chondrocytes from patients

with osteoarthritis. *Mol Med Rep.* 2016 Feb;13(2):1795-800. doi: 10.3892/mmr.2015.4720. Epub 2015 Dec 28.

99. Tang AC, Tang SF, Hong WH, Chen HC. Kinetics features changes before and after intra-articular hyaluronic acid injections in patients with knee osteoarthritis. *Clin Neurol Neurosurg.* 2015 Feb;129 Suppl 1:S21-6. doi: 10.1016/S0303-8467(15)30007-X.

100. Raeissadat SA, Rayegani SM, Hassanabadi H, Fathi M, Ghorbani E, Babaee M, Azma K.Knee Osteoarthritis injection choices: platelet- rich plasma (PRP) versus hyaluronic acid (a one-year randomized clinical trial). *Clin Med Insights Arthritis Musculoskelet Disord.* 2015 Jan 7;8:1-8. doi: 10.4137/CMAMD.S17894. eCollection 2015.

101. Sánchez M, Fiz N, Azofra J, et al. A randomized clinical trial evaluating plasma rich in growth factors (PRGF-Endoret) versus hyaluronic acid in the short-term treatment of symptomatic knee osteoarthritis.. *Arthroscopy.* 2012 Aug;28(8):1070-8.

102. Spaková T, Rosocha J, Lacko M, Harvanová D, Gharaibeh A. Treatment of knee joint osteoarthritis with autologous platelet-rich plasma in comparison with hyaluronic acid. *Am J Phys Med Rehabil.* 2012 May;91(5):411-7.

103. Marx RE et al. Platelet-rich plasma: Growth factor enhancement for bone grafts., *Oral Surg Oral Med Oral Pathol Oral Radiol Endod.,* 1998 Jun;85(6):638-646.

104. Intra-articular hyaluronic acid injection: not for gonarthrosis. *Prescrire Int.* 2013; 22 (142): 248-249.

105. Song YD, Jain NP, Kim S, Kwon SK, Chang MJ, Chang CB, Kim TK. Is knee magnetic resonance imaging overutilized in current practice? *Knee Surg Relat Res.* 2015 Jun;27(2):95-100. doi: 10.5792/ksrr.2015.27.2.95. Epub 2015 Jun 1.

106. Sladjan T, Zoran V, Zoran B. Correlation of clinical examination, ultrasound sonography, and magnetic resonance imaging findings with arthroscopic findings in relation to acute and chronic lateral meniscus injuries. *J Orthop Sci.* 2013 Oct 19.

107. Yanagisawa S, Ohsawa T, Saito K, Kobayashi T, Yamamoto A, Takagishi K. Morphological evaluation and diagnosis of medial type osteoarthritis of the knee using ultrasound. *J Orthop Sci.* 2014 Jan 6.

108. Cellár R, Sokol D, Lacko M, et al. Magnetic resonance imaging in the diagnosis of intra-articular lesions of the knee. *Acta Chir Orthop Traumatol Cech.* 2012;79(3):249-54.

109. Ibid.

110. Wick MC, Jaschke W, Klauser AS. Radiological imaging of osteoarthritis of the knee. *Radiologe.* 2012 Oct 7.

111. Ben-Galim P, Steinberg EL, Amir H, Ash N, Dekel S, Arbel R. Accuracy of magnetic resonance imaging of the knee and unjustified surgery. *Clin Orthop Relat Res.* 2006 Jun;447:100-4.

112. Davatchi F, Sadeghi Abdollahi B, Mohyeddin M, Nikbin B. Mesenchymal stem cell therapy for knee osteoarthritis: 5 years follow-up of three patients. *Int J Rheum Dis.* 2015 May 20. doi: 10.1111/1756-185X.12670. [Epub ahead of print.]

113. Qi Y, Yan W. Mesenchymal stem cell sheet encapsulated cartilage debris provides great potential for cartilage defects repair in osteoarthritis. *Med Hypotheses*. 2012 Sep;79(3):420-1. Epub 2012 Jun 1.

114. Titorencu I, Pruna V, Jinga VV, Simionescu M. Osteoblast ontogeny and implications for bone pathology: an overview. *Cell Tissue Res*. 2014 Jan;355(1):23-33. doi: 10.1007/s00441-013-1750-3. Epub 2013 Nov 29.

115. Calori GM, Mazza E, Colombo M, Mazzola S, Mineo GV, Giannoudis PV. Treatment of AVN using the induction chamber technique and a biological-based approach: Indications and clinical results. *Injury*. 2013 Sep 19. pii: S0020-1383(13)00423-3. doi: 10.1016/j.injury.2013.09.014.

116. Huang S, Xu L, Zhang Y, Sun Y, Li G. Systemic and local administration of allogeneic bone marrow derived mesenchymal stem cells promotes fracture healing in rats. *Cell Transplant*. 2015;24(12):2643-55. doi: 10.3727/096368915X687219. Epub 2015 Feb 2.

117. Kanchanatawan W et al. Short-term outcomes of platelet-rich plasma injection for treatment of osteoarthritis of the knee. *Knee Surg Sports Traumatol Arthrosc*. 2015 Sep 19.

118. Pourcho AM, Smith J, Wisniewski SJ, Sellon JL. Intraarticular platelet-rich plasma injection in the treatment of knee osteoarthritis: review and recommendations. *Am J Phys Med Rehabil*. 2014 Nov;93(11 Suppl 3):S108-21. doi: 10.1097/PHM.0000000000000115.

119. Lyras D et al. Immunohistochemical study of angiogenesis after local administration of platelet rich plasma in a patellar tendon defect. *Intl Orthopaedics* 2010;34(1).

120. Halpern B, Chaudhury S, Rodeo SA, Hayter C, Bogner E, Potter HG, Nguyen J. Clinical and MRI outcomes after platelet-rich plasma treatment for knee osteoarthritis. *Clin J Sport Med*. 2012 Dec 12. [Epub ahead of print.]

121. Oryan A, Alidadi S, Moshiri A. Platelet-rich plasma for bone healing and regeneration. *Expert Opin Biol Ther*. 2016;16(2):213-32. doi: 10.1517/14712598.2016.1118458. Epub 2015 Dec 4.

122. Hirzinger C, Tauber M, Korntner S, Quirchmayr M, Bauer HC, Traweger A, Tempfer H. ACL injuries and stem cell therapy. *Arch Orthop Trauma Surg*. 2014 Nov;134(11):1573-8. doi: 10.1007/s00402-014-2060-2. Epub 2014 Jul 30.

123. Reported by Deren Bagsby, MD, George Gantsoudes, MD, and Robert Klitzman, MD. *Am J Orthop*. 2015;44(8):E294-E297.

124. https://www.hss.edu/newsroom_young-acl-surgery-patients-need-second-surgery.asp

125. Grote W, Delucia R, Waxman R, Zgierska A, Wilson J, Rabago D. Repair of a complete anterior cruciate tear using Prolotherapy: a case report. *Int Musculoskelet Med*. 2009 Dec 1;31(4):159-165.

126. Reeves KD, Hassanein KM. Long-term effects of dextrose Prolotherapy for anterior cruciate ligament laxity. *Altern Ther Health Med*. 2003 May-Jun;9(3):58-62.

127. Franz EW, Bentley JN, Yee PP, Chang KW, Kendall-Thomas J, Park P, Yang LJ. Patient misconceptions concerning lumbar spondylosis diagnosis and

treatment. *J Neurosurg Spine.* 2015 May;22(5):496-502. doi: 10.3171/2014.10. SPINE14537. Epub 2015 Feb 27.

128. Steinberger J, Skovrlj B, Caridi JM, Cho SK. The top 100 classic papers in lumbar spine surgery. *Spine* (Phila. Pa 1976). 2015 May 15;40(10):740-7. doi: 10.1097/BRS.0000000000000847.

129. Wassenaar M, van Rijn RM, van Tulder MW, et al. Magnetic resonance imaging for diagnosing lumbar spinal pathology in adult patients with low back pain or sciatica: a diagnostic systematic review. *Eur Spine J.* 2012 Feb;21(2):220-7. Epub 2011 Sep 16.

130. Steinberger J, Skovrlj B, Caridi JM, Cho SK. The top 100 classic papers in lumbar spine surgery. *Spine* (Phila. Pa 1976). 2015 May 15;40(10):740-7. doi: 10.1097/BRS.0000000000000847.

131. Steffens D, Hancock MJ, Maher CG, Williams C, Jensen TS, Latimer J. Does magnetic resonance imaging predict future low back pain? A systematic review. *Eur J Pain.* 2013 Nov 26. doi: 10.1002/j.1532-2149.2013.00427.x.

132. Balagué F, Dudler J. [Imaging in low back pain: limits and reflexions.] *Rev Med Suisse.* 2013 Jun 26;9(392):1351-2, 1354-6, 1358-9.

133. Emery DJ et al. Overuse of magnetic resonance imaging. *JAMA Intern Med.* 2013 May 13;173(9):823-5. Doi: 10.1001/jamainternmed.2013.3804.

134. Srinivas SV, Deyo RA, Berger ZD. Application of "less is more" to low back pain. *Arch Intern Med.* 2012;172(11):1-5. Doi:10.1001/archinternmed.2012.1838.

135. Andersen JC. Is immediate imaging important in managing low back pain? *J Athl Train.* 2011 Jan-Feb;46(1):99-102.

136. Decision making in surgical treatment of chronic low back pain: the performance of prognostic tests to select patients for lumbar spinal fusion. *Acta Orthop Suppl.* 2013 Feb;84(349):1-35. doi: 10.3109/17453674.2012.753565.

137. Shaffrey CI, Smith JS. Editorial: Stabilization of the sacroiliac joint. *Neurosurg Focus.* 2013 Jul;35(2 Suppl):Editorial. doi: 10.3171/2013.V2.FOCUS13273.

138. el Barzouhi A, Vleggeert-Lankamp CL, Lycklama à Nijeholt GJ, Van der Kallen BF, van den Hout WB, Koes BW, Peul WC; Leiden-Hague Spine Intervention Prognostic Study Group. Predictive value of MRI in decision making for disc surgery for sciatica. *J Neurosurg Spine.* 2013 Dec;19(6):678-87. doi: 10.3171/2013.9.SPINE13349. Epub 2013 Oct 18.

139. Rupert MP, Lee M, Manchikanti L, Datta S, Cohen SP. Evaluation of sacroiliac joint interventions: a systematic appraisal of the literature. *Pain Physician.* 2009 Mar-Apr;12(2):399-418.

140. Hansen H, Manchikanti L, Simopoulos TT, Christo PJ, Gupta S, Smith HS, Hameed H, Cohen SP. A systematic evaluation of the therapeutic effectiveness of sacroiliac joint interventions. *Pain Physician.* 2012 May-Jun;15(3):E247-78.

141. Verrills P, Nowesenitz G, Barnard A. Prevalence and characteristics of discogenic pain in tertiary practice: 223 consecutive cases utilizing lumbar discography. *Pain Med.* 2015 Aug;16(8):1490-9. doi: 10.1111/pme.12809. Epub 2015 Jul 27.

142. Ellingson AM, Shaw MN, Giambini H, An KN. Comparative role of disc

degeneration and ligament failure on functional mechanics of the lumbar spine. *Comput Methods Biomech Biomed Engin.* 2015 Sep 24;1-10.

143. Romero-Vargas S. Profile of the patient with failed back surgery syndrome in the National Institute of Rehabilitation. Comparative analysis. *Cir.* 2015 Mar-Apr;83(2):117-23. doi:10.1016/j.circir.2015.04.006. Epub 2015 May 16. PubMed 10.1016/j.circir.2015.04.006. Epub 2015 May 16.

144. Bhatia A, Flamer D, Shah PS, Cohen SP. Transforaminal epidural steroid injections for treating lumbosacral radicular pain from herniated intervertebral discs: a systematic review and meta-analysis. *Anesth Analg.* 2016 Mar;122(3):857-70. doi: 10.1213/ANE.0000000000001155.

145. Leung SM et al. Clinical value of transforaminal epidural steroid injection in lumbar radiculopathy. *Hong Kong Med J.* 2015 Aug 14. doi: 10.12809/hkmj144310

146. Zarghooni K, Rashidi A, Siewe J, Röllinghoff M, Bredow J, Eysel P, Scheyerer MJ. Single-shot epidural injections in the management of radicular pain. *Orthop Rev (Pavia).* 2015 Dec 28;7(4):5985. doi: 10.4081/or.2015.5985. eCollection 2015 Dec 28. PubMed PMID: 26793292; PubMed Central PMCID: PMC4703910.

147. Radcliff K, Hilibrand A, Lurie JD, Tosteson TD, Delasotta L, Rihn J, Zhao W, Vaccaro A, Albert TJ, Weinstein JN. The impact of epidural steroid injections on the outcomes of patients treated for lumbar disc herniation: a subgroup analysis of the SPORT trial, *J Bone Joint Surg Am.* 2012 Jun 27. doi: 10.2106/JBJS.K.00341. [Epub ahead of print.]

148. Epstein NE. The risks of epidural and transforaminal steroid injections in the spine: commentary and a comprehensive review of the literature. *Spine.* 2013;3:74-93.

149. Stout A. Epidural steroid injections for low back pain. *Phys Med Rehabil Clin N Am.* 2010 Nov;21(4):825-34.

150. Svensson GL, Lundberg M, Ostgaard HC, Wendt GK. High degree of kinesiophobia after lumbar disc herniation surgery. *Acta Orthop.* 2011 Dec;82(6):732-6. Epub 2011 Nov 9.

151. Rundell SD, Davenport TE. Patient education based on principles of cognitive behavioral therapy for a patient with persistent low back pain: a case report. *J Orthop Sports Phys Ther.* 2010;40(8):494–501. doi:10.2519/jospt.2010.3264.

152. Archer KR, Devin CJ, Vanston SW, Cognitive-behavioral based physical therapy for patients with chronic pain undergoing lumbar spine surgery: a randomized controlled trial. *J Pain.* 2015 Oct 14. pii: S1526-5900(15)00906-2. doi: 10.1016/j.jpain.2015.09.013

153. Deyo RA, Martin BI, Kreuter W, Jarvik JG, Angier H, Mirza SK. Revision surgery following operations for lumbar stenosis. *J Bone Joint Surg Am.* 2011 Nov 2;93(21):1979-86.

154. Martin BI, Mirza SK, Comstock BA, Gray DT, Kreuter W, Deyo RA. Reoperation rates following lumbar spine surgery and the influence of spinal fusion procedures. *Spine* (Phila. Pa 1976). 2007 Feb 1;32(3):382-7.

155. Röllinghoff M, Schlüter-Brust K, Groos D, et al. Mid-range outcomes in 64 consecutive cases of multilevel fusion for degenerative diseases of the lumbar spine. *Orthop Rev* (Pavia). 2010;2(1):e3. doi:10.4081/or.2010.e3.

156. Von Forell GA, Stephens TK, Samartzis D, Bowden AE. Low back pain: A biomechanical rationale based on "patterns" of disc degeneration. *Spine* (Phila. Pa 1976). 2015 May 20.

157. Gullung GB1, Woodall JW, Tucci MA, James J, Black DA, McGuire RA. Platelet-rich plasma effects on degenerative disc disease: analysis of histology and imaging in an animal model. *Evid Based Spine Care J.* 2011 Nov;2(4):13-8. doi: 10.1055/s-0031-1274752.

158. Khalaf K, Nikkhoo M, Ya-Wen Kuo, Yu-Chun Hsu, Parnianpour M, Campbell-Kyureghyan N, Haghpanahi M, Jaw-Lin Wang. Recovering the mechanical properties of denatured intervertebral discs through Platelet-Rich Plasma therapy. *Conf. Proc. IEEE Eng. Med. Biol. Soc.* 2015 Aug; 2015:933-6. doi: 10.1109/EMBC.2015.7318516.

159. O'Shea FD, Boyle E, Salonen DC, Ammendolia C, Peterson C, Hsu W, Inman RD. Inflammatory and degenerative sacroiliac joint disease in a primary back pain cohort. *Arthritis Care Res.* (Hoboken). 2010 Apr;62(4):447-54. doi: 10.1002/acr.20168.

160. Umapathy H, Bennell K, Dickson C, Dobson F, Fransen M, Jones G, Hunter DJ. The web-based osteoarthritis management resource my Joint pain improves quality of care: a quasi-experimental study. *J Med Internet Res.* 2015 Jul 7;17(7):e167. doi: 10.2196/jmir.4376.

161. Stacey D, Taljaard M, Dervin G, Tugwell P, O'Connor AM, Pomey MP, Boland L, Beach S, Meltzer D, Hawker G. Impact of patient decision aids on appropriate and timely access to hip or knee arthroplasty for osteoarthritis: a randomized controlled trial. *Osteoarthritis Cartilage.* 2016 Jan;24(1):99-107. doi: 10.1016/j.joca.2015.07.024. Epub 2015 Aug 4.

162. Selten EM, Vriezekolk JE, Geenen R, van der Laan WH, van der Meulen-Dilling RG, Nijhof MW, Schers HJ, van den Ende CH. Reasons for treatment choices in knee and hip osteoarthritis: A qualitative study. *Arthritis Care Res.* (Hoboken). 2016 Jan 27. doi: 10.1002/acr.22841

163. Pitta M, Davis W, Argintar EH. Arthroscopic Management of Osteoarthritis. *J Am Acad Orthop Surg.* 2016 Feb;24(2):74-82. doi: 10.5435/JAAOS-D-14-00258.

164. Keeney JA, Nunley RM, Adelani M, Mall N. Magnetic resonance imaging of the hip: poor cost utility for treatment of adult patients with hip pain. *Clin Orthop Relat Res.* 2014 Mar;472(3):787-92. doi: 10.1007/s11999-013-3431-7. Epub 2013 Dec 21.

165. Tasoglu O, Sirzai H, Onat SS, Ozgirgin N. Is hip originated pain misdiagnosed? *Pain Physician.* 2015 Mar-Apr;18(2):E259-60.

166. van Zyl AA. Misdiagnosis of hip pain could lead to unnecessary spinal surgery. *SA Orthop J* (Pretoria). 2010; 9(4).

167. Ferrata P, Carta S, Fortina M, Scipio D, Riva A, Di Giacinto S. Painful hip arthroplasty: definition. *Clin Cases Miner Bone Metab.* 2011 May;8(2):19-22.

168. Abbas K, Murtaza G, Umer M, Rashid H, Qadir I. Complications of total hip replacement. *J Coll Physicians Surg Pak.* 2012 Sep;22(9):575-8. doi: 09.2012/JCPSP.575578.

169. Panegrossi G, Ceretti M, Papalia M, Casella F, Favetti F, Falez F. Bone loss management in total knee revision surgery. *Int Orthop.* 2014 Jan 10

170. Hernigou P, Flouzat-Lachaniette CH, Delambre J, Poignard A, Allain J, Chevallier N, Rouard H. Osteonecrosis repair with bone marrow cell therapies: state of the clinical art. *Bone.* 2014 Jul 10. pii: S8756-3282(14)00257-9. doi: 10.1016/j.bone.2014.04.034.

171. Lau RL, Perruccio AV, Evans HM, Mahomed SR, Mahomed NN, Gandhi R. Stem Cell Therapy for the treatment of early stage avascular necrosis of the femoral head: a systematic review. *BMC Musculoskelet Disord.* 2014 May 16;15:156. doi: 10.1186/1471-2474-15-156.

172. Houdek MT, Wyles CC, Martin JR, Sierra RJ. Stem cell treatment for avascular necrosis of the femoral head: current perspectives. *Stem Cells Cloning.* 2014 Apr 9;7:65-70. eCollection 2014.

173. Bottai V, Dell'Osso G, Celli F, Bugelli Gi, Cazzella N, Cei E, Guido G, Giannotti S. Total hip replacement in osteoarthritis: the role of bone metabolism and its complications. *Clin Cases Miner Bone Metab.* 2015 Sep-Dec;12(3):247-50. doi: 10.11138/ccmbm/2015.12.3.247. Epub 2015 Dec 29.

174. Civinini R, Nistri L, Martini C, Redl B, Ristori G, Innocenti M. Growth factors in the treatment of early osteoarthritis. *Cli. Cases Miner Bone Metab.* 2013 Jan;10(1):26-9. doi: 10.11138/ccmbm/2013.10.1.026. PubMed Abstract.

175. Sánchez M, Guadilla J, Fiz N, Andia I. Ultrasound-guided platelet-rich plasma injections for the treatment of osteoarthritis of the hip. *Rheumatology* (Oxford). 2012 Jan;51(1):144-50.

176. Dallari D, Stagni C, Rani N, Sabbioni G, Pelotti P, Torricelli P, Tschon M, Giavaresi G. Ultrasound-guided injection of platelet-rich plasma and hyaluronic acid, separately and in combination, for hip osteoarthritis: a randomized controlled study. *Am. Sports Med.* 2016 Jan 21. pii: 0363546515[620383].

177. Emadedin M, Ghorbani Liastani M, Fazeli R, Mohseni F, et al. Long-term follow-up of intra-articular injection of autologous mesenchymal stem cells in patients with knee, ankle, or hip osteoarthritis. *Arch Iran Med.* 2015 Jun;18(6):336-44. doi: 015186/AIM.003.

178. Fouilleron N, Wavreille G, Endjah N, et al. Running activity after hip resurfacing arthroplasty: a prospective study. *Am J Sports Med.* 2012 Apr;40(4):889-94. doi: 10.1177/0363546511434564. Epub 2012 Feb 1.

179. Le Duff MJ, Amstutz HC. The relationship of sporting activity and implant survivorship after hip resurfacing. *J Bone Joint Surg Am.* 2012 May 16;94(10):911-8.

180. Smith MV, Costic RS, Allaire R, Schilling PL, Sekiya JK. A biomechanical analysis of the soft tissue and osseous constraints of the hip joint. *Knee Surg Sports Traumatol Arthrosc.* 2012 Oct 30.

181. Lin DJ, Wong TT, Kazam JK. Shoulder Arthroplasty, from indications to complications: what the radiologist needs to know. *Radiographics.* 2016 Jan-Feb;36(1):192-208. doi: 10.1148/rg.2016150055.

182. Ansari F, Lee T, Malito L, Martin A, Gunther SB, Harmsen S, Norris TR, Ries M, Van Citters D, Pruitt L. Analysis of severely fractured glenoid components: clinical consequences of biomechanics, design, and materials selection on implant performance. *J Shoulder Elbow Surg.* 2016 Jan 14. pii: S1058-2746(15)00588-1. doi: 10.1016/j.jse.2015.10.017

183. Knowles NK, Ferreira LM, Athwal GS. The arthritic glenoid: anatomy and arthroplasty designs. *Curr Rev Musculoskelet Med.* 2016 Jan 23.

184. Cisneros LG, Atoun E, Abraham R, Tsvieli O, Bruguera J, Levy O. Revision shoulder arthroplasty: does the stem really matter? *J. Shoulder Elbow Surg.* 2016 Jan 25. pii: S1058-2746(15)00578-9. doi: 10.1016/j.jse.2015.10.007.

185. Mei-Dan O, Carmont MR. The role of platelet-rich plasma in rotator cuff repair. *Sports Med Arthrosc.* 2011 Sep;19(3):244-50.

186. Banke IJ, Vogt S, Buchmann S, Imhoff AB. [Arthroscopic options for regenerative treatment of cartilage defects in the shoulder]. *Orthopäde.* 2011 Jan;40(1):85-92. doi: 10.1007/s00132-010-1682-5.

187. Craig EV, Galatz LM, Sperling JW. From platelet-rich plasma to the reverse prosthesis: controversies in treating rotator cuff pathology. *Instr Course Lect.* 2014;63:63-70.

188. Keener JD, Galatz LM, Teefey SA, et al. A prospective evaluation of survivorship of asymptomatic degenerative rotator cuff tears. *J Bone Joint Surg Am.* 2015 January;97(2):89-98. doi:10.2106/JBJS.N.00099.

189. Garbis NG, McFarland EG. Understanding and evaluating shoulder pain in the throwing athlete. *Phys Med and Rehabil Clinics of North Am.* 2014; 25 (4): 735. doi:10.1016/j.pmr.2014.06.009.

190. von Wehren L, Blanke F, Todorov A, Heisterbach P, Sailer J, Majewski M. The effect of subacromial injections of autologous conditioned plasma versus cortisone for the treatment of symptomatic partial rotator cuff tears. *Knee Surg Sports Traumatol Arthrosc.* 2015 May 28. [Epub ahead of print.]

191. Valencia Mora M, Ruiz Ibán MA, Díaz Heredia J, Barco Laakso R, Cuéllar R, García Arranz M. Stem cell therapy in the management of shoulder rotator cuff disorders. *World J Stem Cells.* 2015 May 26;7(4):691-9. doi: 10.4252/wjsc.v7.i4.691.

192. Brockmeyer M, Tompkins M, Kohn DM, Lorbach O. SLAP lesions: a treatment algorithm. *Knee Surg Sports Traumatol Arthrosc.* 2016 Feb;24(2):447-55. doi: 10.1007/s00167-015-3966-0. Epub 2016 Jan 27.

193. A worrisome trend in SLAP repair. AAOS. http://www.aaos.org/AAOSNow/2010/Aug/clinical/clinical2/?ssopc=1

194. Tashjian RZ. Is there evidence in favor of surgical interventions for the subacromial impingement syndrome? *Clin J Sport Med.* 2013 Sep;23(5):406-7. doi: 10.1097/01.jsm.0000433152.74183.53.

195. Castagna A, Delle Rose G, Borroni M, Cillis BD, Conti M, Garofalo R, Ferguson D, Portinaro N. Arthroscopic stabilization of the shoulder in adolescent athletes participating in overhead or contact sports. *Arthroscopy.* 2012 Mar; 28(3):309-15. doi: 10.1016/j.arthro.2011.08.302. Epub 2011 Nov 30.

196. Strauss EJ, McCormack RA, Onyekwelu I, Rokito AS. Management of failed

arthroscopic rotator cuff repair. *J Am Acad Orthop Surg.* 2012 May;20(5):301-9.

197. Lee DH, Kwack KS, Rah UW, Yoon SH. Prolotherapy for refractory rotator cuff disease: retrospective case-control study of 1-year follow-up. *Arch Phy. Med Rehabil.* 2015 Aug 5. pii: S0003-9993(15)00594-8. doi: 10.1016/j.apmr.2015.07.011.

198. von Wehren L, Blanke F, Todorov A, Heisterbach P, Sailer J, Majewski M. The effect of subacromial injections of autologous conditioned plasma versus cortisone for the treatment of symptomatic partial rotator cuff tears. *Knee Surg Sports Traumatol Arthrosc.* 2015 May 28.

199. Mei-Dan O, Carmont MR. The role of platelet-rich plasma in rotator cuff repair. *Sports Med Arthrosc.* 2011 Sep;19(3):244-50.

200. Yadav R, Kothari SY, Borah D. Comparison of local injection of platelet-rich plasma and corticosteroids in the treatment of lateral epicondylitis of humerus. *J Clin Diagn Res.* 2015 Jul;9(7):RC05-7. doi: 10.7860/JCDR/2015/14087.6213.

201. Arirachakaran A, Sukthuayat A, Sisayanarane T, Laoratanavoraphong S, Kanchanatawan W, Kongtharvonskul J. Platelet-rich plasma versus autologous blood versus steroid injection in lateral epicondylitis: systematic review and network meta-analysis. *J Orthop Traumatol.* 2015 Sep 11.

202. Gosens T, Peerbooms JC, van Laar W, den Oudsten BL. Ongoing positive effect of platelet-rich plasma versus corticosteroid injection in lateral epicondylitis: a double-blind randomized controlled trial with 2-year follow-up. *Am J Sports Med.* 2011 Jun;39(6):1200-8. Epub 2011 Mar 21.

203. Dong W, Goost H, Lin XB, Burger C, Paul C, Wang ZL, Kong FL, Welle K, Jiang ZC, Kabir K. Injection therapies for lateral epicondylalgia: a systematic review and Bayesian network meta-analysis. *Br J Sports Med.* 2015 Sep 21. pii: bjsports-2014-094387. doi: 10.1136/bjsports-2014-094387.

204. Murray DJ, Javed S, Jain N, Kemp S, Watts AC. Platelet-rich-plasma injections in treating lateral epicondylosis: a review of the recent evidence. *J Hand Microsurg.* 2015 Dec;7(2):320-5. doi: 10.1007/s12593-015-0193-3. Epub 2015 Jul 8.

205. Kahlenberg CA, Knesek M, Terry MA. New developments in the use of biologics and other modalities in the management of lateral epicondylitis. *BioMed Res Int.* Volume 2015 (2015), Article ID 439309. http://dx.doi.org/10.1155/2015/439309

206. Degenerative cervical spine disease may not progress over time. *Newswise.* http://www.newswise.com/articles/degenerative-cervical-spine-disease-may-not-progress-over-time

207. Helgeson MD, Albert TJ. Surgery for failed cervical spine reconstruction. *Spine* (Phila. Pa 1976). 2011 Nov 8. [Epub ahead of print.]

208. Fu MC, Webb ML, Buerba RA, et al. Comparison of agreement of cervical spine degenerative pathology findings in magnetic resonance imaging studies. *Spine J.* 2016 Jan 1;16(1):42-8. doi: 10.1016/j.spinee.2015.08.026. Epub 2015 Aug 17.

209. Centeno CJ, Elliott J, Elkins WL, Freeman M. Fluoroscopically guided cervical Prolotherapy for instability with blinded pre and post radiographic reading.. *Pain Physician.* 2005;8:67-72.

210. Myrtveit SM, Skogen JC, Sivertsen B, et al. Pain and pain tolerance in whiplash-associated disorders: a population-based study. *Eur J Pain*. 2015 Nov 16. doi: 10.1002/ejp.819. [Epub ahead of print.]

211. Vernon H, Guerriero R, Kavanaugh S, Puhl A. Is "fear of passive movement" a distinctive component of the Fear-Avoidance Model in whiplash? *J Can Chiropr Assoc*. 2015 Sep;59(3):288-93.

212. Casey PP, Feyer AM, Cameron ID. Course of recovery for whiplash associated disorders in a compensation setting. *Injury*. 2015 Nov;46(11):2118-29. doi: 10.1016/j.injury.2015.08.038. Epub 2015 Sep 3.

213. Hegab AF et al. Platelet-rich plasma injection as an effective treatment for temporomandibular joint osteoarthritis. *J Oral Maxillofac Surg*. 2015 Sep;73(9):1706-13. doi: 10.1016/j.joms.2015.03.045. Epub 2015 Mar 24.

214. Hancı M, Karamese M, Tosun Z, Aktan TM, Duman S, Savaci N. Intra-articular platelet-rich plasma injection for the treatment of temporomandibular disorders and a comparison with arthrocentesis. *J Craniomaxillofac Surg*. 2015 Jan;43(1):162-6. doi: 10.1016/j.jcms.2014.11.002. Epub 2014 Nov 15.

215. Pihut M, Szuta M, Ferendiuk E, Zeńczak-Więckiewicz D. Evaluation of pain regression in patients with temporomandibular dysfunction treated by intra-articular platelet-rich plasma injections: a preliminary report. *Biomed Res Int*. 2014;2014:132369. doi: 10.1155/2014/132369. Epub 2014 Aug 3.

216. Refai H, Altahhan O, Elsharkawy R. The efficacy of dextrose Prolotherapy for temporomandibular joint hypermobility: a preliminary prospective, randomized, double-blind, placebo-controlled clinical trial. *J Oral Maxillofac Surg*. 2011 Dec;69(12):2962-70. Epub 2011 Jul 16.

217. He M, Gan AW, Lim AY, Goh JC, Hui JH, Chong AK. Bone marrow derived mesenchymal stem cell augmentation of rabbit flexor tendon healing. *Hand Surg*. 2015 Oct;20(3):421-9. doi: 10.1142/S0218810415500343. PubMed.

218. Tetta C, Consiglio AL, Bruno S, Tetta E, Gatti E, Dobreva M, Cremonesi F, Camussi G. The role of microvesicles derived from mesenchymal stem cells in tissue regeneration; a dream for tendon repair? *Muscles Ligaments Tendons J*. 2012 Oct 16;2(3):212-21. Print 2012 Jul.

219. Shapiro E, Grande D, Drakos M. Biologics in Achilles tendon healing and repair: a review. *Curr Rev Musculoskelet Med*. 2015 Feb 6. PubMed.

220. Gosens T, Den Oudsten BL, Fievez E, van't Spijker P, Fievez A. Pain and activity levels before and after platelet-rich plasma injection treatment of patellar tendinopathy: a prospective cohort study and the influence of previous treatments. *Int Orthop*. 2012 Apr 27. [Epub ahead of print.]

221. von Wehren L, Blanke F, Todorov A, Heisterbach P, Sailer J, Majewski M. The effect of subacromial injections of autologous conditioned plasma versus cortisone for the treatment of symptomatic partial rotator cuff tears. *Knee Surg Sports Traumatol Arthrosc*. 2015 May 28.

222. Valencia Mora M, Ruiz Ibán MA, Díaz Heredia J, Barco Laakso R, Cuéllar R, García Arranz M. Stem cell therapy in the management of shoulder rotator cuff disorders. *World J Stem Cells*. 2015 May 26;7(4):691-9. doi: 10.4252/wjsc.v7.i4.691.

223. López-Gavito E, Gómez-Carlín LA, Parra-Téllez P, Vázquez-Escamilla J. Platelet-rich plasma for managing calcaneus tendon tendinopathy and plantar fasciitis. *Acta Ortop Mex.* 2011 Nov-Dec;25(6):380-5. PubMed PRP Abstract.

224. Gaweda K, Tarczynska M, Krzyzanowski W. Treatment of Achilles tendinopathy with platelet-rich plasma. *Int J Sports Med.* 2010 Aug;31(8):577-83. Epub 2010 Jun 9. PubMed Abstract.

225. Guelfi M, Pantalone A, Vanni D, Abate M, et al. Long-term beneficial effects of platelet-rich plasma for non-insertional Achilles tendinopathy. Foot Ankle Surg. 2015 Sep;21(3):178-81. doi: 10.1016/j.fas.2014.11.005. Epub 2014 Dec 11. PUBMED ABSTRACT

226. Zheng H, Chen C. Body mass index and risk of knee osteoarthritis: systematic review and meta-analysis of prospective studies. *BMJ Open.* 2015 Dec 11;5(12):e007568. doi: 10.1136/bmjopen-2014-007568.

227. Collins KH, Hart DA, Reimer RA, Seerattan RA, Herzog W. Response to diet-induced obesity produces time-dependent induction and progression of metabolic osteoarthritis in rat knees. *J Orthop Res.* 2016 Jun;34(6):1010-8.. doi: 10.1002/jor.23103.

228. Giuseppe Musumeci et al. Osteoarthritis in the XXIst century: risk factors and behaviours that influence disease onset and progression. *Int J Mol Sci.* 2015 Mar; 16(3): 6093–6112. PubMed.

229. Bray GA,Smith SR, de Jonge L, et al. Effect of dietary protein content on weight gain, energy expenditure, and body composition during overeating: a randomized controlled trial. *JAMA* 2012;307(1):47-55. doi: 10.1001/jama.2011.1918.

230. Weiss EP, Racette SB, Villareal DT, Fontana L, Steger-May K, Schechtman KB, Klein S, Ehsani AA, Holloszy JO. Lower extremity muscle size and strength and aerobic capacity decrease with caloric restriction but not with exercise-induced weight loss. *J Appl Physiol.* 2007 Feb;102(2):634-40. Epub 2006 Nov 9.

231. Hussain SM, Cicuttini FM, Giles GG, Graves SE, Wang Y. Relationship between circulating sex steroid hormone concentrations and incidence of total knee and hip arthroplasty due to osteoarthritis in men. *Osteoarthritis Cartilage.* 2016 Apr 12. pii: S1063-4584(16)30024-3. doi: 10.1016/j.joca.2016.04.008. [Epub ahead of print.]

232. Almehmadi Y, Yassin AA, Nettleship JE, Saad F. Testosterone replacement therapy improves the health-related quality of life of men diagnosed with late-onset hypogonadism. *Arab J Urol.* 2016 Mar;14(1):31-6. doi: 10.1016/j.aju.2015.10.002. Epub 2015 Nov 27.

233. Cepeda MS, Zhu V, Vorsanger G, Eichenbaum G. Effect of opioids on testosterone levels: cross-sectional study using NHANES. *Pain Med.* 2015 Dec;16(12):2235-42. doi: 10.1111/pme.12843. PubMed.

234. Bawor M, Bami H, Dennis B, et al. Testosterone suppression in opioid users: a systematic review and meta-analysis. *Drug Alcohol Depend.* 2015 Apr 1;149:1-9. doi: 10.1016/j.drugalcdep.2015.01.038. Epub 2015 Feb 8.

235. Bawor M et al. Testosterone suppression in opioid users: a systematic review

and meta-analysis. *Drug Alcohol Depend.* 2015 Feb 8. pii: S0376-8716(15)00073-3. doi: 10.1016/j.drugalcdep.2015.01.038. [Epub ahead of print.]

236. Basaria S. Effects of testosterone replacement in men with opioid-induced androgen deficiency: a randomized controlled trial. *Pain.* 2015 Feb;156(2):280-8. doi: 10.1097/01.j.pain.0000460308.86819.aa.

237. Tennant F. Hormone abnormalities in patients with severe and chronic pain who fail standard treatments. *Postgrad Med.* 2015 Jan;127(1):1-4. Epub 2014 Dec 15.

238. Kobara M, Furumori-Yukiya A, Kitamura M, Matsumura M, Ohigashi M, Toba H, Nakata T. Short-term caloric restriction suppresses cardiac oxidative stress and hypertrophy from chronic pressure overload. *J Card Fail.* 2015 May 13. pii: S1071-9164(15)00127-X. doi: 10.1016/j.cardfail.2015.04.016. [Epub ahead of print.]

239. Yokokawa T, Sato K, Iwanaka N, Honda H, Higashida K, Iemitsu M, Hayashi T, Hashimoto T. Dehydroepiandrosterone activates AMP kinase and regulates GLUT4 and PGC-1α expression in C2C12 myotubes. *Biochem Biophys Res Commun.* 2015 May 15. pii: S0006-291X(15)00908-0. doi: 10.1016/j.bbrc.2015.05.013. [Epub ahead of print.]

240. Gong H, Han YW, Sun L. The effects of energy intake of four different feeding patterns in rats. *Exp Biol Med* (Maywood). 2015 May 12. pii: 1535370215584890. [Epub ahead of print.]

241. Yanai H, Toren D, Vierlinger K, Hofner M, Nöhammer C, Chilosi M, Budovsky A, Fraifeld VE. Wound healing and longevity: lessons from long-lived αMUPA mice. *Aging* (Albany, NY). 2015 Mar;7(3):167-76. [Erratum: *Aging* 2016.]

242. Wu S. Fasting triggers stem cell regeneration of damaged, old immune system. *USC News.* 2014 June 5. http://news.usc.edu/63669/fasting-triggers-stem-cell-regeneration-of-damaged-old-immune-system

243. Testa G, Biasi F, Poli G, Chiarpotto E. Calorie restriction and dietary restriction mimetics: a strategy for improving healthy aging and longevity. *Curr Pharm Des.* 2013 Sep 26. [Epub ahead of print.]

244. Bhanot S, Alex JC. Current applications of platelet gels in facial plastic surgery. Current applications of platelet gels in facial plastic surgery. Facial Plast Surg. 2002 Feb; 18(1):27-33.

245. Man D, Plosker H, Winland-Brown JE. The use of autologous platelet-rich plasma (platelet gel) and autologous platelet-poor plasma (fibrin glue) in cosmetic surgery. Plast Reconstr Surg. 2001 Jan; 107(1):229-37; discussion 238-9.

246. Fitzpatrick RE, Rostan EF. Reversal of photodamage with topical growth factors: a pilot study. J Cosmet Laser Ther. 2003 Apr;5 (1):25-34.

247. Abuaf OK, Yildiz H, Baloglu H, Bilgili ME, Simsek HA, Dogan B. Histologic Evidence of New Collagen Formulation Using Platelet Rich Plasma in Skin Rejuvenation: A Prospective Controlled Clinical Study. Annals of Dermatology. 2016; 28(6):718-724. doi:10.5021/ad.2016.28.6.718.

248. Lu Y.Effects of "surrounding needling" on hydroxyproline content and ultra-

structures in the dermis of aged rats. Zhongguo Zhen Jiu. 2008 Jan; 28(1):61-4.

249. Sclafani AP, McCormick SA. Induction of dermal collagenesis, angiogenesis, and adipogenesis in human skin by injection of platelet-rich fibrin matrix. Arch Facial Plast Surg. 2012 Mar-Apr;14(2):132-6. doi: 10.1001/archfacial.2011.784. Epub 2011 Oct 17.

250. Redaelli A, Romano D, Marcianó A. Face and neck revitalization with platelet-rich plasma (PRP): clinical outcome in a series of 23 consecutively treated patients. J Drugs Dermatol. 2010 May; 9(5):466-72.

251. Yuksel EP, Sahin G, Aydin F, Senturk N, Turanli AY. Evaluation of effects of platelet-rich plasma on human facial skin. J Cosmet Laser Ther. 2014 Oct;16(5): 206-8. doi: 10.3109/14764172.2014.949274. Epub 2014 Aug 25.

252. Cervelli, Valerio MD; Lucarini, Lucilla MD.Use of Platelet-Rich Plasma and Hyaluronic Acid in the Loss of Substance with Bone Exposure. Advances in Skin & Wound Care: April 2011 - Volume 24 - Issue 4 - pp 176-181

253. Ulusal BG. Platelet-rich plasma and hyaluronic acid—an efficient biostimulation method for face rejuvenation. J Cosmet Dermatol. 2016 Sep 5. doi: 10.1111/jocd.12271.

254. Pei M, Zhang Y, Li J, Chen D. Antioxidation of decellularized stem cell matrix promotes human synovium-derived stem cell-based chondrogenesis. Stem Cells Dev. 2013 Mar 15; 22(6):889-900. doi: 10.1089/scd.2012.0495. Epub 2012 Dec 16.

255. Nofal E, Helmy A, Nofal A, Alakad R, Nasr M. Platelet-rich plasma versus CROSS technique with 100% trichloroacetic acid versus combined skin needling and platelet rich plasma in the treatment of atrophic acne scars: a comparative study. Dermatol Surg. 2014 Aug; 40(8):864-73.

256. Khatu SS, More YE, Gokhale NR, Chavhan DC, Bendsure N. Platelet-Rich Plasma in Androgenic Alopecia: Myth or an Effective Tool. Journal of Cutaneous and Aesthetic Surgery. 2014;7(2):107-110. doi:10.4103/0974-2077.138352.

257. Gupta AK, Carviel J. A Mechanistic Model of Platelet-Rich Plasma Treatment for Androgenetic Alopecia. Dermatol Surg. 2016 Dec;42(12):1335-1339.

258. Maria-Angeliki G, Alexandros-Efstratios K, Dimitris R2, Konstantinos K. Platelet-rich Plasma as a Potential Treatment for Noncicatricial Alopecias. Int J Trichology. 2015 Apr-Jun;7(2):54-63. doi: 10.4103/0974-7753.160098.

259. Singhal P, Agarwal S, Dhot PS, Sayal SK. Efficacy of platelet-rich plasma in treatment of androgenic alopecia. Asian J Transfus Sci. 2015 Jul-Dec;9(2):159-62. doi: 10.4103/0973-6247.162713.

260. Gkini MA, Kouskoukis AE, Tripsianis G, Rigopoulos D, Kouskoukis K. Study of platelet-rich plasma injections in the treatment of androgenetic alopecia through an one-year period. J Cutan Aesthet Surg. 2014 Oct-Dec;7(4):213-9. doi: 10.4103/0974-2077.150743.

261. Khatu SS, More YE, Gokhale NR, Chavhan DC, Bendsure N. Platelet-Rich Plasma in Androgenic Alopecia: Myth or an Effective Tool. Journal of Cutaneous and Aesthetic Surgery. 2014;7(2):107-110. doi:10.4103/0974-2077.138352.

262. Singhal P, Agarwal S, Dhot PS, Sayal SK. Efficacy of platelet-rich plasma in treatment of androgenic alopecia. Asian J Transfus Sci. 2015 Jul-Dec;9(2):159-62. doi: 10.4103/0973-6247.162713.

263. El Taieb MA, Ibrahim H, Nada EA, Seif Al-Din M. Platelets rich plasma versus minoxidil 5% in treatment of alopecia areata: A trichoscopic evaluation. Dermatol Ther. 2017 Jan;30(1). doi: 10.1111/dth.12437. Epub 2016 Oct 28.

264. Gentile P1, Garcovich S2, Bielli A3, Scioli MG3, Orlandi A3, Cervelli V4. The Effect of Platelet-Rich Plasma in Hair Regrowth: A Randomized Placebo-Controlled Trial. Stem Cells Transl Med. 2015 Nov;4(11):1317-23. doi: 10.5966/sctm.2015-0107. Epub 2015 Sep 23.

Index

Page references in *italics* denote photographs or figures.

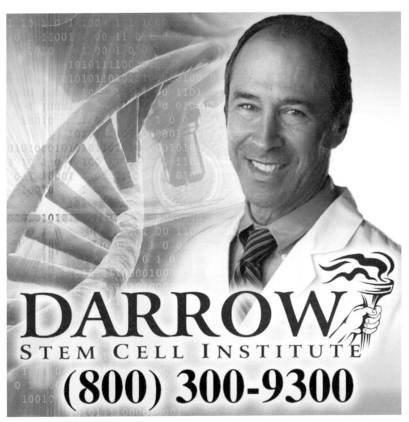

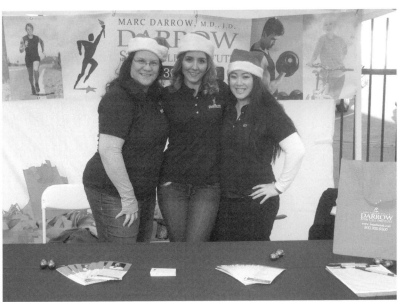

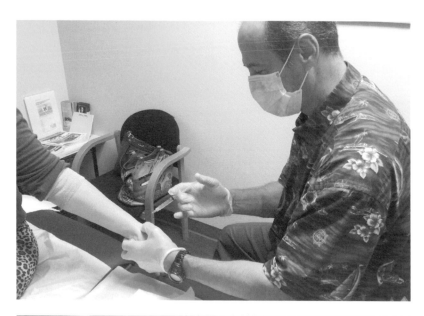

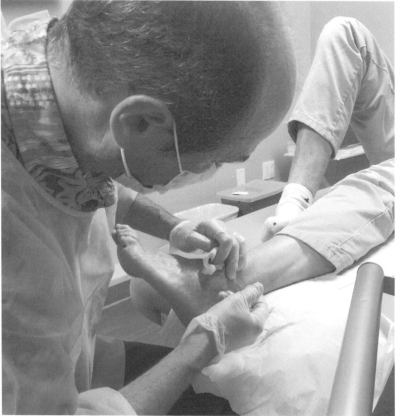

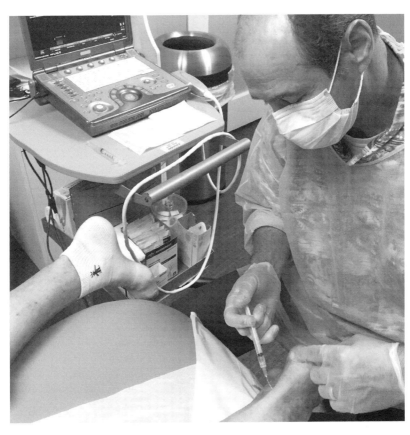

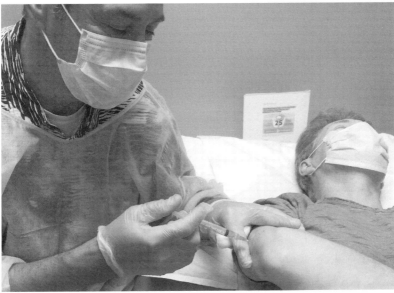

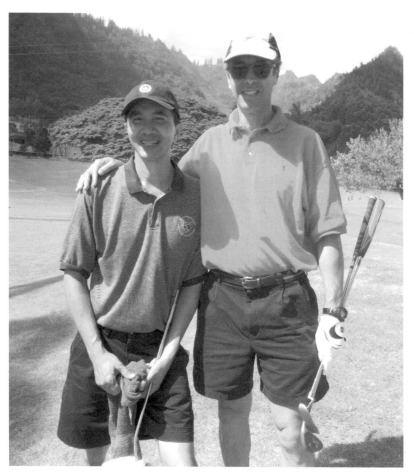

Hawaii

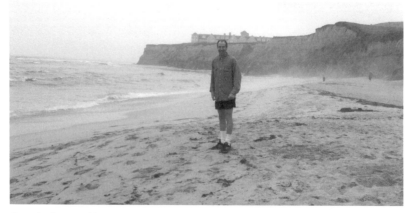

Ritz-Carlton, Half Moon Bay

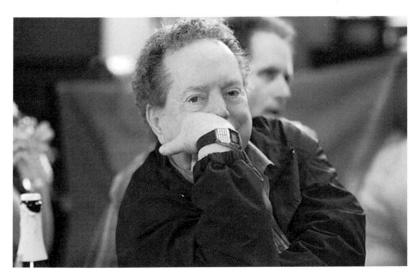

John-Roger

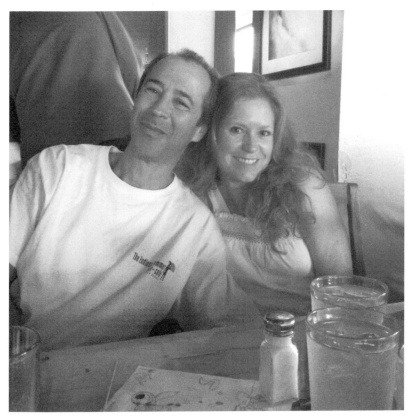

Marc and Michelle Darrow

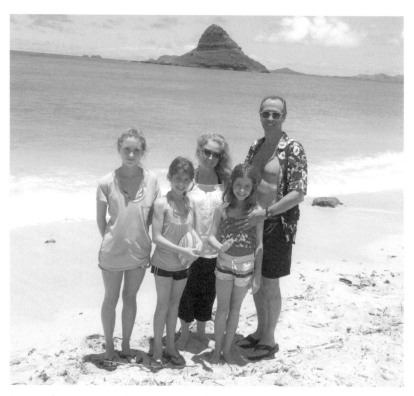

Darrow family in Hawaii at Chinaman's Hat

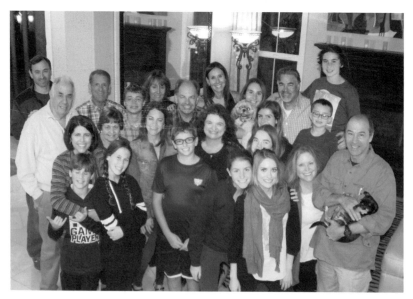

Darrow family Thanksgiving